D0742444

TRAUMA AND ADOLESCENCE

Monograph Series

of the International Society for

Adolescent Psychiatry

Volume 1

Trauma and Adolescence

edited by

Max Sugar, M.D.

International Universities Press, Inc.
Madison   Connecticut

Library of Congress Cataloging-in-Publication Data

Trauma and adolescence / edited by Max Sugar.
    p.   cm. — (Monograph series of the Society for Adolescent Psychiatry ; v. 1)
  Includes bibliographical references and indexes.
  ISBN 0-8236-6626-3
  1. Psychic trauma in adolescence.   I. Sugar, Max, 1925-   .
II. Series.
RJ506.P66T73   1999
616.85'21'00835—dc21   98-52743
                                                  CIP

Manufactured in the United States of America

Contents

Preface

With the launching of this monograph series the International Society for Adolescent Psychiatry moves into another phase of its continuing development.

The idea of the monographs arose from various lengthy discussions about the need to focus on a particular topic and bring new insights to that area. The International Society for Adolescent Psychiatry provides the possibility for sharing, comparing, and learning about both normative development, and the prevention and treatment of pathology in adolescence in different cultures around the world. The multinational aspects add to the special appeal of this psychiatric society and also of the monographs.

This first volume, on *Trauma and Adolescence,* consists of three sections: Psychoanalytic Aspects; The Trauma of Physical and Psychosomatic Illness; and Social Disruption and the Adolescent Process. Although the topic of trauma in adolescence has by no means been exhausted, by examining it from the psychoanalytic, somatic, and societal viewpoints as it pertains to adolescence, the volume illuminates special areas needing further attention.

Samuel Rubin focuses on the effects of psychic trauma on adolescent ego organization in his chapter on "Trauma in Adolescence: Psychoanalytic Perspectives." He points out that with early childhood trauma and pathological interactions a faulty foundation is set up that makes the youngster vulnerable to difficulties in emotional functioning in adolescence.

Paola Carbone and Eleda Spano consider "Trauma as a Potential Psychic Organizer" in adolescence. Their hypothesis challenges the exclusivity of viewing trauma only as negative, and suggests that trauma may also serve as an organizer involving the nucleus of the adolescent's condition. The trauma establishes inner contact with some split-off and isolated pathological parts of the self which have previously been occluded. In therapy, which brings these together, the youngster may then move on to improved functioning and involvement with the environment.

Gunther Perdigao writes on "Mourning in Children and Adolescents" and discusses whether mourning is possible in children. He provides clinical material derived from the analysis of a child in latency, and his second analysis as an adolescent. He demonstrates the presence of continuing conflict and shows that analytic work is subject to reversal following further massive trauma. With the second analysis the patient was able to consider his original feelings about his mother's death, and work successfully on the issue of mourning.

In "The Psychodrama of Trauma and the Trauma of Psychodrama," Maja Perret-Catipovic and François Ladame recommend the use of individual psychoanalytic psychodrama with multiple therapists who participate in the drama along with the adolescent patient. They find that this is a very beneficial approach when the adolescent's treatment is mired despite efforts to deal with the resistance, or when the youngster is inhibited and avoidant with apparent confusion between internal and external reality.

In the section on physical and psychosomatic illness, the focus is on the effects of physical conditions from which children would not have survived in the past. This reflects advances in medicine and the challenges provided by survival against high odds.

In "The Separation–Individuation Process in Adolescents with Chronic Physical Illness," Magda Liakopoulou points out that separation-individuation is impeded due to illness, the narcissistic trauma caused by the illness, and the lowering of self-esteem. She presents case material to illustrate this, and also focuses on the psychiatrist's approach to treatment in such situations.

In her chapter on "Difficulties Encountered by Adolescent Thalassemia Patients," Dionysia Panitz notes that this condition affects the whole family and has especially serious repercussions in the mother–child relationship. If he or she lives through adolescence, the thalassemia patient has demanding developmental tasks to face which are intensified by anxiety, denial, and regression, due to the prolonged and difficult course of the illness. The most severe crises occur when the diagnosis is first made, and then in adolescence.

Sylvie Pucheu, Paola Antonelli, and Silla Consoli observe that the psychodynamic processes in adolescence, and those involved in the emotional integration of a kidney graft, seem to be similar in their effects on the reorganization of the body image, the acceptance of a new image, and the reactivation of castration anxiety and the oedipus complex. An interesting thesis is developed about the coping issues involved in a successful integration of a transplanted organ.

Margaret Stuber and Anne Kazak provide a view of "The Developmental Impact of Cancer Diagnosis and Treatment for Adolescents." Whilst they discuss developmental consequences that are, to some extent, negative, they also point out there may be some positive benefits to the survivor of childhood or adolescent cancer having to do with an appreciation of life and a different perspective on values.

In the section on societal disruption, James Garbarino focuses on "What Children Can Tell Us about Living with Violence." He feels that such children need help to recover from their experiences, but that emotionally disabled or immobilized adults seem unlikely to provide it. An important message of safety is needed from the adults for them to be seen as havens of protection and authority for such children.

Max Sugar's chapter on "Severe Physical Trauma in Adolescence" focuses on the cognitive, emotional, physical, and behavioral aspects of adolescents involved in physical trauma. The effects are detailed along with the various behaviors and problems in recognition and obtaining treatment.

Honig, Grace, Lindy, Newman, and Titchener describe the long-term effects of disasters occurring during childhood and adolescence. They note that children's and adolescents' sensibilities are crushed during catastrophes by the impact of chaos and proximity to death, all of which imprint loss and devastation on their surroundings. Following the initial crisis there is reorganization of the self, the family, the community, and the socioeconomic systems, with varying effects. Their chapter presents ongoing research on the Buffalo Creek disaster.

David Rothstein's chapter focuses on "Lethal Identity: Violence and Identity Formation," and the issue of the leader performing particular functions for followers by providing help in the regulation of their self-esteem. People select self-objects, items of a public nature, to become part of their self-system. The successful leader recognizes these self-objects and elevates the followers' self-object. The leader makes himself available as an object of identification, and his or her particular personal characteristics interact with contemporary historic events which determine how well the leader performs these functions for the followers. In this situation the population gets the kind of leader it is seeking. Rothstein provides illustrations of this concept by referring both to historical figures and patients.

Annette Streeck-Fischer provides further amplification of this theme from the side of the follower, with her chapter on "Xenophobia and Violence by Adolescent Skinheads." She indicates that the violent environment of the extreme right offers male youths a specific kind of stability which supports their adolescent self-system while simultaneously intensifying personality malformations. She presents some case histories which illustrate her concept that through the processes of adaptation and assimilation there develops a grandiose self, a peer ideology, and a self-reparative transformation of self-hatred into xenophobia with a regressive sexual desire that becomes a lust for violence.

The final chapter by Max Sugar discusses "Adolescent Survivors of the Holocaust." It appears that their development was arrested, and they had incomplete mourning. Alongside this there were countertransference issues in evaluating and treating these survivors, which included difficulties in making a diagnosis consistent with the facts of their situation.

Acknowledgments

In the process of parturition and delivery of the first offspring in the series, some significant help was provided by a number of diligent attendants. First, I mention with great pleasure, the continued support of Dr. Michael Kalogerakis, the president of the International Society for Adolescent Psychiatry. The stimulation and support given by the late Dr. Joseph Noshpitz in his capacity as coordinator of publications was invaluable. Drs. Irving H. Berkovitz, Remi Gonzalez, Gerald Wiener, and Jacob M. Weisler assisted by their review of some papers. Last, but not least, the continued and untiring efforts of my secretary, Mrs. Dora V. Posey, need to be emphasized.

Contributors

Paola Antonelli, Ph.D., is on the faculty of the Department of Liaison Psychiatry and Medical Psychology, Broussais Hospital, Paris, France.

Paola Carbone, M.D., is Assistant Professor, Development and Socialization Department, University of Rome "La Sapienza," Rome, Italy.

Silla M. Consoli, M.D., is Professor of Psychiatry, Department of Liaison Psychiatry and Medical Psychology, Broussais Hospital, Paris, France.

James Garbarino, Ph.D., is Director, Family Life Development Center; Professor, Human Development, Cornell University, Ithaca, New York.

Mary C. Grace, M.Ed., M.S., is Senior Research Associate, Department of Psychiatry, University of Cincinnati College of Medicine, Cincinnati, Ohio.

Richard G. Honig, M.D., is Training and Supervising Analyst, Cincinnati Psychoanalytic Institute; Assistant Clinical Professor of Psychiatry, University of Cincinnati College of Medicine, Department of Psychiatry, Cincinnati, Ohio.

Anne E. Kazak, Ph.D., is Director, Psychosocial Services, Division of Oncology, The Children's Hospital of Philadelphia; Associate Professor of Pediatrics and Psychiatry, University of Pennsylvania School of Medicine, Philadelphia, Pennsylvania.

François Ladame, M.D., is on the faculty of the Department of Psychiatry, Geneva University Hospitals, Faculty of Medicine, University of Geneva, Geneva, Switzerland.

Magda Liakopoulou, M.D., is Director, Consultation-Liaison Child Psychiatry, Child Psychiatry Department, Aghia Sofia Children's Hospital, Athens, Greece.

Jack D. Lindy, M.D., is Training and Supervising Analyst, and Director, Cincinnati Psychoanalytic Institute, Cincinnati, Ohio.

C. Janet Newman, M.D., is Professor Emeritus of Psychiatry and Child Psychiatry, University of Cincinnati College of Medicine; Faculty, Cincinnati Psychoanalytic Institute, Cincinnati, Ohio.

Dionysia Panitz, Dipl.Psych., is on the faculty of the Department of Psychological Pediatrics, Aghia Sophia Children's Hospital, Athens, Greece.

H. Gunther Perdigao, M.D., is Training and Supervising Analyst, Child and Adult, New Orleans Psychoanalytic Institute, New Orleans, Louisiana.

Maja Perret-Catipovic, M.A., is on the faculty of the Unité de Psychiatrie de l'Adolescence, Department of Psychiatry, Faculty of Medicine, University of Geneva, Switzerland.

Sylvie Pucheu, Ph.D., is on the faculty of the Department of Psychiatry and Medical Psychology, Broussais Hospital, Paris, France.

David A. Rothstein, M.D., is in private practice in Chicago.

Samuel E. Rubin, M.D., is Clinical Professor of Psychiatry, Louisiana State School of Medicine and Tulane University School of Medicine, New Orleans; Training and Supervising Analyst, Child and Adult, New Orleans Psychoanalytic Institute, New Orleans, Louisiana.

Eleda Spano, M.A., Dott.Psychol., is on the faculty of the Department of Neurosciences Development, University of Rome, Rome, Italy.

Annette Streeck-Fischer, M.D., is Chief of Child Psychiatry and Psychotherapy, Tiefenbrunn Hospital, Tiefenbrunn, Germany; Training Analyst Lou Andreas-Salome Institute of Psychoanalysis and Psychotherapy, Gottingen; Lecturer at University Medical School of Gottingen, Herzberger, Germany.

Margaret L. Stuber, M.D., is Associate Professor, Department of Psychiatry, University of California at Los Angeles.

Max Sugar, M.D., is Clinical Professor of Psychiatry, Louisiana
State University, School of Medicine and Tulane University
School of Medicine, New Orleans, Louisiana.

James L. Titchener, M.D., is Professor Emeritus of Psychiatry,
University of Cincinnati College of Medicine; Training and
Supervising Analyst, Cincinnati Psychoanalytic Institute, Cin-
cinnati, Ohio.

Part I

Psychoanalytic Aspects

1

Trauma in Adolescence

Psychoanalytic Perspectives

Samuel E. Rubin, M.D.

The combination of adolescence and trauma brings together two areas, each of which involves complex issues. Adolescence is a phase of development that has varying degrees of stress, and offers the child a chance for a major restructuring of his or her personality. When the experience of trauma is added during the adolescent period and/or earlier in childhood, with either positive or negative effects for development, we can see the multitude of potential alterations and forces impinging on the child's mind and personality.

The Phases of Adolescence

In the process of becoming an adolescent the child enters a psychological era in which the upsurge in the drives along with oedipal conflicts can lead to regressive conflicts with parents. There ensues the progressive detachment from these parental objects and an increasing investment in peers and the discovery of adults

3

in the outside world who can serve as ideals. The struggle in progressive development is frequently expressed as a conflict between idealizing these adults and disappointment at finding them "hypocritical," or having feet of clay. The superego temporarily loses its functional structure as the adolescent lets go of his or her parents and attempts to integrate a more personal conscience. This can lead to occasional delinquent acts or a seeming loss of values and standards. Increased anxiety and conflict with the parents may augment the stress already present in the family.

The increased drive pressures, an admixture of sexual and aggressive, are expressed in masturbatory activity with its accompanying fantasies. The fantasies include sadomasochistic, homosexual, and heterosexual themes which in most cases in middle and late adolescence gradually become heterosexual with objects from the adolescent's real world. Sometimes heroic grandiose fantasies develop which defend against the anxieties of the adolescent's independence and autonomy. Relationships and thoughts of the future, including fantasies of marriage and career, become part of the adolescent's day and night dreams.

REVIEW OF THE LITERATURE

The notion of trauma as presented here conceptualizes it as a relative idea based on a number of variables. These include the individual's adolescent vulnerability or resistance to sudden, unexpected traumatic overstimulation which, however brief, overwhelms the ego and produces a state of helplessness. One individual might experience a traumatic overstimulation while another might not be so affected (Rangell, 1967). Fatigue, illness, or exhaustion may make the adolescent more vulnerable to a particular stimulus. The early life experiences of the adolescent, and how he or she coped with inner and outer stimuli, have a bearing on vulnerability during adolescence. Trauma in early childhood, especially early preoedipal trauma, sensitizes the youngster to the repetition of trauma during the adolescent passage, as Greenacre (1967) has pointed out. Early trauma such as the illness, death, and loss of a parent or sibling, or sexual overstimulation, and/or abuse may predispose the adolescent to repeated traumatic experiences. The experience becomes sexualized, that is, linked with internal libidinal fantasies. Although some authors, including Rangell (1967), address the notion of trauma from an external quantitative and qualitative point of view, the effect of an incident is a matter of speculation. I believe that the traumatic potential of a real life incident rests with its inner psychic effect to produce a state of overwhelming anxiety and partial or total ego disintegration and disorganization. This effect may be inferred by the observer. The extent of the trauma-induced helplessness at times can only be assessed through understanding the individual's inner experience. Trauma from the infantile period may result in ego restriction and avoidance which creates increased tensions and difficulty for the restructuring experiences of adolescence. Trauma may have a negative effect, with the emergence of neurotic symptoms, or may have a positive effect which facilitates ego defense and adaptation. As an example, an adolescent being seen for anxiety symptoms had an almost fatal automobile accident. He returned to therapy and announced that he was discontinuing his therapy since his survival and coping with the momentary overwhelming fear for his life made his ordinary anxiety "ridiculous" by comparison.

The concept of trauma was introduced by Freud in *Studies on Hysteria* (Breuer and Freud, 1893–1895) when he considered sexual traumas to be the result of real seductions. Only later did Freud recognize the conflictual potential of inner fantasies. In 1920 he proposed the concept of the stimulus barrier, which represents the ego defenses that provide protection from overstimulation. Initially, the mother's ego serves as a protection against overwhelming stimulation. A combination of endowment and experience, the complemental series, determines an element of vulnerability to traumatic overstimulation. Freud's addition to the definition of trauma in 1926 continues to be useful, namely, a sudden overwhelming stimulation that immobilizes the ego functions and results in a state of helplessness. The delimiting of the concept enables us to better study trauma, compare our data, and understand its effects. As A. Freud (1967) states, it enables us to differentiate trauma from pathological factors. She points out that there are two characteristics of trauma: (1) its suddenness, which does not allow for defensive shifts; and (2) some immediate aftereffect indicating ego disruption. Furst (1967a) emphasizes that the regression is not only a reaction to the flood of anxiety, but an adaptive attempt to master and bind the tension. Greenacre (1967) adds to the concept of trauma her clinical experience that the most profound effects of trauma occur in the preoedipal period between the ages of 2 and 4 and can never be digested; that is, the individual is prone to breakdown. By these definitions an outer, real, and potentially traumatic event may become traumatic to the ego if the event touches upon inner anxieties or wishful fantasies. This is in line with Furst's thinking that when overt traumatic experiences touch upon underlying fantasies, there is a greater tendency for fixation of the conflict. For a more extensive discussion of the historical development of the analytic perspective on trauma see Breuer and Freud (1893–1895), Freud (1920, 1926), and Furst's *Psychic Trauma* (1967b), especially the articles by Furst (1967a), Rangell (1967), Greenacre (1967), and A. Freud (1967).

A more recent contribution by Sandler, Dreher, and Drews (1991) introduced a paradigm for psychoanalytic research. The premise utilized is that of a group of analysts discussing their concepts of psychic trauma. Through their discussions preconscious concepts emerged that are contributory to psychoanalytic theory building. From their discussions there were four categories for organizing the study of trauma: (1) the traumatic situation, understood as the links between the event and the experience; (2) the consequences of the traumatic situation; (3) the predisposition to being traumatized; and (4) the implications for therapeutic technique. There were differing emphases in considering what is traumatic. Some thought the event had to have subjective significance for the individual. Some weighted internal factors, such as drive-related invested fantasies which could overwhelm the individual from within, and thus result in a traumatic state of helplessness. In considering the consequences of trauma, there was thought to be first, the immediate psychic wound, and second, the aftereffects, which include an active conflict, or as I conceptualize it, a fixation that is prone to erupt in conflict and symptoms given the appropriate stimulus. The fixation of a traumatic incident produces ripples in the personality that lead to adaptive and defensive struggles. These produce a wide variety of possible symptoms and character traits, some adaptive and some maladaptive, leading to deformations of the individual's personality. I will now present two clinical examples that illustrate some of the factors that were mentioned previously.

CASE ILLUSTRATION 1

The first patient, Ms. B, was an attractive 15-year-old who appeared for her first appointment in a state of turmoil. She rambled in a confused, agitated way, speaking of the death six weeks earlier of her best friend's father, and her friend's subsequent move from the city. Ms. B spoke of her infatuation with a boy named Art, to which she associated in clang fashion with an art course at school. A concurrent dental infection and the recommendation for oral surgery weighed heavily upon her. As she rambled on she would occasionally curse, "shit," and giggle. My comment acknowledging her upset brought forth a reply that she felt she was talking in a "dream" and felt "drunk." After three sessions, Ms. B spontaneously became coherent, and the agitation and giggling abated. She reported once again being able to sleep, after a month of insomnia. Additional data from later in the treatment revealed that Ms. B had a congenital shortening of the toes of her right foot. She also had urinary retention, and a hesitancy to use any bathroom other than at home.

Ms. B was the "baby" of a lower middle-class Catholic family, which included an older brother and two older sisters. She attended a Catholic girl's school where she was in the 10th grade. Ms. B was an A student on partial scholarship. The parents noted that she worried about grades and was a perfectionist. The father was an articulate, hard-working mechanic who had completed high school. Ms. B's mother appeared to be an insensitive, guilty woman who spoke in a loud, anxious voice. Only later was I to learn that the mother was partially deaf, and resisted wearing a hearing aid. The maternal grandmother and grandfather had lived in the home from B's birth until their simultaneous deaths, when she was $8^1/2$ to 9. Until two to three years earlier, she had refused to go to sleep by herself.

In considering her personality development and the current psychopathology, I struggled to understand the nature of the diagnosis and hence the treatment of choice. It seemed that her ego functioning was disorganized and she had a psychotic condition. Perhaps there had been a schizophrenic process underlying what seemed to be a previous good adaptation and ego functioning, and she now had a schizophrenic disorder. There was ample evidence for object loss which included the deaths of the grandparents and her best friend's father, as well as the loss of her friend due to a move. She had experienced anxiety prior to this acute episode and yet had relationships, was bright, an academic achiever, and psychologically minded. Her conflicts seemed to center around sexual issues, the body anxiety stirred up by the threat of dental surgery, and rather severe superego guilt. The sudden onset of her disorganizing anxiety, of short duration once she was seen (three visits), and the premorbid development, pointed to a hysterical character structure and a hysterical neurosis. (I was reminded of Zetzel's [1968]) paper on "The So-Called Good Hysteric.") I therefore recommended intensive analytic therapy four times weekly. Our work terminated after four-and-one-half years.

In considering the interface between this young adolescent girl's personality structure and trauma, it would be useful to sketch out in some detail how the trauma of the death of her girl friend's father interdigitated with her early conflicts, especially the early fixations. The opening themes centered around her feelings that men are better than women. She brought in a diary for me to read which clearly showed her conflicts over her sexual desires and her religious–moral ideas. She found these difficult to verbalize. This was linked to two screen memories: one at age 3, of father watching her on the toilet; and the second, at age 8, of seeing a man masturbating in a car. Her difficulty verbalizing seemed to be related to a transference feeling that she would be supervised too closely and criticized, which reminded her of her mother. Her defenses were highlighted in a dream illustrating the dynamics of the anal withholding silences and her attempts to launder out uncomfortable sexual material.

Ms. B's contemplation of dental surgery was accompanied by a transference experience in the office when she suddenly experienced "turning cold." She associated to her silences and to her operation as a "manicure" which she also saw as the analytic operation of wanting to be male, and feeling she was a second-class citizen as a female. The sense I had at the time was that we had a good alliance and that we could work together to understand her feelings of being defective as a girl. The work indeed proceeded well as we worked on the bisexual conflicts and her identification with her father. The analyst's first vacation was met with fears that something might happen to him, an accident or death. These associations reminded me that her girl friend's father's death had been a precipitant of the psychotic episode leading to her therapy. Little work could be done with this since her denial increased and the material shifted. My attempts to engage her in understanding her reactions to the separation were met with teasing and mocking responses.

B elaborated her feelings of being defective as she recalled her fear at the onset of her menses at age 13. She did not know where the blood was coming from, and was fearful of finding out (i.e., looking). As we worked with her fear and her defenses against looking, and the holding back silences, she shared a dream with oedipal associations and themes of sibling rivalry: "Father with a gun. Someone shoots my sister in the front room."

She reported another dream indicating her hostile rivalry with her mother: "My mother is dead. I wake up crying and I can't stop."

Following these dreams, we came to understand her mocking and teasing of the analyst as a defensive identification with her father. I had a feeling that we were working well together and that she was making good use of the therapy. I was to be surprised later by the extent and rapidity of her regression.

We worked on a pregnancy fantasy in which the woman is the active phallic one while the man is receptive. B fantasized she had lost her birthstone ring in the toilet and was angry that her mother had never replaced it. I heard this as a reference to her idea of having lost a phallus. As she worked on the issues of her penis envy, self-damage, anal loss, and anger at her mother, and as the analyst's vacation approached, marking the end of our second year of work, she expressed a fantasy of graduating from the analysis. Exploration of this fantasy led to our understanding that she was not ready to finish, but that it represented a defense against looking further. This was accompanied by a series of disaster dreams which included themes from well-known movies such as the *Poseidon Adventure*.

She contemplated going through with the dental surgery. The death of her paternal grandmother at this time increased her fear of the stormy voyage of the therapy. As B approached her rage at her sense of damage (castration), penis envy, and separation fears, she experienced increasing anxiety and helplessness over losing control. Her presenting symptoms reappeared. I recommended she sit up face-to-face, after having used the couch throughout the analysis. This was intended to enhance her reality testing and to slow the overwhelming anxiety and the regressive disorganization she was experiencing. Attempts to help her to integrate the emerging fear and rage toward the analyst–mother failed. Memories of anal seductive trauma with increasing projection and homosexual anxiety became overwhelming. Because of her ego disorganization and open threats to kill her mother and her mother's masochistic response of "go ahead," hospitalization was recommended and readily accepted. B was hospitalized by another psychiatrist, and within three weeks she had reintegrated on no medication and was discharged. She returned to therapy in the third week of her hospitalization and continued using the couch thereafter.

B's motivation to understand her disorganization was impressive. She was able to verbalize the hostile transference, expressing anger at the analyst for not understanding her, not being ready to stop the analysis, and her wish for rescue by the analyst. She shared her mistrust of the analyst and her secret fear of going crazy. Material centering around separation-individuation and her feminine identity were articulated clearly as she expressed the feeling that she was glued to the couch, that is, the therapist. As a child she could never leave without screaming and temper tantrums. Her rage at being a woman and not a man was expressed in her secret wish that she could be anything and that analysis would make her a man. B openly stated, "Why else did I come here, but to get what I lost?" She felt so tortured by these feelings of helpless anger and disappointment that she wanted to torture and defeat the analyst. She realized that these two issues were covered by two main defenses as she conceptualized them. These were first, a filing system in her mind in which some of the filed things got misplaced and lost (repressions), and second, an image of an overflowing toilet, the recent psychotic episode which represented projection and expulsion.

The therapeutic alliance was now quite solid and we could proceed to understand what had happened. Central to this was the exploration and elaboration of the hostile identification with her mother, "momma rat," a nickname given the mother by the father. B was angry with her father for the rejection and the devaluation of her mother and herself.

We could see the fear of her sexuality as she associated to the analyst's summer vacation. Three fantasies emerged which became focal points for the therapeutic work. She fantasized (1) the analyst was married with three kids; (2) no, he was just queer; and (3) no, he's fooling around and might take me to the mountains for a new experience. B's sense of incompleteness as a woman was expressed in a more integrated way prior to the vacation. "Women aren't equipped the way a man is, so you don't think that way"; that is, a woman is weak and unprepared for separations. The analysis proceeded over the next two-and-one-half years to a termination without another psychotic episode. I will describe some of the difficulties of this ending process later.

The major themes of this treatment have been outlined. This adolescent girl's difficulties, as demonstrated, centered around separation and abandonment, and her ambivalent fusion with her mother. However, oedipal themes and conflicts on all levels of her development were touched upon. The central difficulty in dealing with object loss and the resulting regression in the face of her traumatic helplessness, brought B to therapy. It surfaced again after two years of intensive analytic work with the death of her paternal grandmother and her defensive desire to leave the analysis. Although I gave B no indication that I agreed with her stopping, and in fact I thought she herself understood this, and was not going to stop, nothing we tried could arrest the severe regressive disorganization that erupted. The difference at the two-year point was our recognition of her profound rage at her mother, which also reflected her hatred of herself as a rat child of her rat mother. I came to learn from the parents that B had had a traumatic first year of life during which she had cried inconsolably. Her mother, ostensibly, could not hear her, and the mother had refused to get a hearing aid. The father expressed his ambivalent, angry devaluation of the mother by calling her "momma rat." This devaluation extended itself to B. B was deprived not only of the comfort and affect modulation by her mother, but also came to feel the hostile rejection of the father. The patient's fantasy of having "a new experience with the analyst, an affair" meant the possibility of having a father who affirmed her femininity, a reparative experience. In the transference, B's feeling that she was "glued to the couch" indicated her fusion with the analyst-mother who would comfort her, and provide her with what she was missing (i.e., a sense of her self-worth as a girl). These difficulties existed not only in my patient, but also in an older sister who also had a transient psychosis, and in an older brother who could never leave the family.

Greenacre (1967) has put forth her idea, gained from her analytic work, that early traumatic experience in the preoedipal period puts a stamp of vulnerability on the ego of the individual. The person is vulnerable to reexperiencing traumatic anxiety which is disorganizing and reproduces a state of helplessness. Historically, B experienced these traumatic states throughout her early years every time she had to separate. She had headaches and stomachaches on leaving home and her mother to go to school. However, she had managed to go to school and be a good girl by toughing it out and defending against her separation fears. The fear that this overwhelming separation anxiety might recur existed for her and me as we worked through her conflicts and approached the termination of her therapy.

Following the reworking of her maternal and paternal identifications, her separation fears, and oedipal fantasies, she mentioned the idea of stopping the analysis. She fantasized it would be like leaving the hospital when the psychiatrist had notified her she would be leaving in eleven days. Since I thought she had worked on her major conflicts I said that when she felt ready we could consider a date which would allow enough time to help her work through her feelings and fantasies of completion.

In the ensuing month B brought in material centering on not wanting to stop, with fears and threats of going "crazy' if the analyst allowed her to terminate. She also reported that six months prior to her recent psychotic episode a male patient of mine had terminated with me, and she feared "I would be next." Although I thought the analysis was proceeding well and anticipated completion of the process when B was ready and with her actively involved, I was apprehensive that the termination period would be a stormy one. I wondered about the possibility of another psychotic episode.

B spontaneously expressed the wish to complete the analysis prior to my vacation. She also reported that she had never been able to say "good-bye,"; "I'm stubborn." Her need to deny my vacation was interpreted in terms of her feelings of sadness and rejection. B's idea also allowed for us to leave together. The date she suggested left us two months to work on her feelings about leaving.

Following this date-setting, B went into a rapid regression, getting "sick," with physical symptoms of stomachaches and openly wishing she were sicker than she was. She canceled a session because she was sick. B recalled a clear oedipal dream that indicated her wish to hang onto the analyst-father by being sick. There followed two sessions in which B sat up facing me saying she was too sick to lie down. Her insomnia returned. Work with her feelings of rejection, affection, and desire to have the analyst control her enabled her to regroup and return spontaneously to the couch. Following this minor storm and continuing therapeutic work, B felt she could now face me and say good-bye.

B was able to express fantasies on all levels of conflict, with affectionate feelings and feelings of rejection being the predominant ones. She felt excited over being independent, and entered driver training. She fantasized both that she would return for monthly checkups, and that she would never see me again. In the last session she was silent and expressed the feeling she had said all she had to say. I thought she feared giving expression to her sad and angry feelings. Six months after our last session, she sent a holiday greeting card with a message which represented the last session. The message was friendly. She was doing well even though she had ups and down. She was going with a boy. She expressed appreciation for the help and how she was a "spoiled brat." B hoped she would become a mature woman. She closed with the idea she had never been able to say good-bye and now wished to say it.

I have presented the course of this young adolescent's therapy in some detail to illustrate the unusual course her treatment took based on the early trauma she had experienced and its effect on her ego. She was especially sensitive to loss and separation which induced profound regression, such as helplessness and disorganization in the face of overwhelming sadness, anger, and object loss. This sensitivity made her vulnerable during her adolescence with the upsurge of the drives and the pressure to detach from her parental objects. The loss of her girl friend's father coincided with her unconscious anger at her own father who devalued her mother and her as females. She also lost the best friend when she moved out of town. B's ego had not been able to modify and integrate, nor develop the capacity to modulate her affects. This I believe was in part due to the mother's unresponsiveness to B's distress in infancy. When most infants are receiving the needed material ego aid and having their needs met, B experienced a flooding of frustration and stimulation that led to a deformation and deficit in her ego functioning. Could analysis and therapy cure or repair this early damage? In this particular girl I believe the answer is no, for I have seen her periodically through the years when she became threatened with loss. She has experienced a powerful need to fuse with someone, a man, and as an example, the analyst. This seems motivated by her need to feel protected from the threat of ego disorganization. Our visits are usually time-limited and she is then able to function on her own. The older brother has never been able to separate from his parents with whom he continues to live.

Case Illustration 2

The second patient, a 12-year-old male, A, was brought for consultation because he was a worrier and an underachiever in school. He was described as too adultlike. A was fearful of riding in elevators and that his parents would die. He experienced nightmares. The fearfulness dated back to his third year of life. The parents were well-educated professionals who were achievers. The father worried that he had hurt his son the way his own father had hurt him. The father had had a destructive relationship with his father which was unresolved. The paternal grandfather was reported by the father to be a hypercritical, intolerant man who never accepted him. He had consciously tried to relate to A in an affectionate, positive way. I was to learn that the father, too, was fearful and carried a gun in his car because he was afraid of "the worst contingencies.'' The mother was a warm woman who had tried to modify her husband's short temper, and also his compulsive need to be with his son, by which he tried to undo his deeply unhappy relationship with his father (paternal grandfather). She was a teacher and focused on her son's underachievement. Of historical significance were the following experiences as related by the youngster in the therapeutic process: (1) At age 2, he had been yelled at by the father for finger painting on the walls in imitation of the father who was painting the house. (2) At age 3, A responded to his mother's screams from the shower during her miscarriage, while the father was out of town. (3) At age 6, his only sibling, a sister, was born. (4) At age 6, a woman friend of the family shot her husband. (5) A series of eight deaths had occurred during his brief lifetime, including friends of his family, and his maternal grandfather.

In assessing him, I thought his anxiety and symptoms were on a neurotic level, with phobic and obsessional features. A had friends, related well, and there were no indications of any reality-testing problem, or psychotic potential. The major source of the distress in the boy was the onset of puberty and adolescent development with the attendant strain on the parental relationships, the increased anxiety of A's relinquishing his parents and becoming independent. How could he deal with his underlying unresolved aggression toward both parents as expressed in his fears that his parents might die? I wondered about his sexual development and how he was dealing with his masturbatory conflicts. There was little data about this initially. I was also unaware at that point of the early trauma that A had experienced at age 3. Since the anxiety symptoms were longstanding, I recommended intensive therapy. He and the parents agreed to twice-a-week sessions.

The initial phase of the work with A centered around his anger and disappointment with his father. This material emerged in the context of his pervasive feeling that his parents were so accomplished that he could never compete with them, much less surpass them. Therefore, if he could not be the best, and better them, he would be the worst. He felt the father pressed him to be with him more than he wanted to be. This served as part of his early resistance to meeting more intensively, and led to his desire to interrupt the therapy after the first year. He complained of his father's overbearing attitude. A had adopted very adultlike behavior in which he tried to participate in the discussions, and listened attentively to all his father's friends as they discussed business ideas. He wanted to learn all he could, and be accepted by adults. After about a year of twice-a-week therapy he announced that he was better and wished to discontinue his treatment. Although I outlined several areas that we had not explored, and interpreted his fear of depending too much on the therapy, A was insistent that he wanted to stop. I agreed. He said he wanted a chance to go on his own and would return if he had difficulties.

About a year later I received a call that A wanted to return. He related that he had wanted to try it on his own and that he was not comfortable being dependent upon me. Shortly after he had interrupted his therapy his maternal grandfather had died. The grandfather had been hemiparetic for many years, and he wondered how his grandmother had dealt with it. Increasingly, he had become depressed, had developed fears of going to sleep, along with suicidal feelings and thoughts. This distress convinced him to return. Based on the seriousness of his growing despair, his fears, and the alliance I thought we had, I recommended that we work intensively, and so we met four times weekly.

A was noticeably different when he returned. The grandiose sense that he could manage everything, and prove he was smarter than his teachers (and adults in general, and his analyst), was no longer evident. Instead, he approached the sessions with a sense that he really wanted to understand himself and relieve his distress. We came to understand that his despair was in part a result of his disappointment that he could not manage his upset and conflicts himself without help. Additionally, he continued to feel that he could not be as accomplished as his parents. The theme of his trying to be so grown-up and self-sufficient continued.

He attended parochial school where he was the leader of a group that rebelled against the religious teachings by challenging the beliefs of the Brothers who were the teachers, and debated the material. He took great pleasure in besting and beating up the teachers with his debate, and basked in the admiration he felt was coming from his group of peers. He enjoyed his ability to manipulate adults. His main activity with his peers was in conducting and participating in role-playing games whose theme was Dracula (connected with the bloody miscarriage) and related characters. He enjoyed his knowledge of the "real" story of Dracula and the misinformation most people had about this. His haughty attitude was a source of irritation for me, and required my self-observation and understanding to not act out my counter-transference. This was part of an enactment in our sessions of his attempting to engage me in debate in which he could best me to prove me helpless and impotent.

As we continued our work his anger clearly surfaced as he "forgot" to put the top up on his father's convertible, which resulted in the car getting soaked. Although A denied that anger with his father was connected with his forgetting, the father's yelling at him repeated the disappointment and helplessness he had experienced as a toddler, and through the years. The early experience of his being yelled at had been passively experienced. His defense of identification with the aggressor had been developed so that he could actively stimulate his father's temper, and then feel superior and in control.

Gradually, his haughty, grandiose attitude gave way to increased anxiety symptoms including psychosomatic nausea, elevator fear, fear of something happening to his parents (they might die), and increasing separation anxiety. This resulted in his being unable to leave home to attend school. His pseudo-adult identity gave way to identity diffusion, and a growing sense of his guilty fears which were based on his "acting" and angry actions, including his precocious sexual behavior, his angry, secret business of stealing his father's liquor and selling it to peers, his selling pornography and feeling he had arranged it so he could not be implicated. He identified with the "Godfather," and his friends were the Mafia family, his distorted, angry ideal. He also identified with Frankenstein's monster, a reflection of his poor self-esteem, and his alienation from his father. The continuing discussion and elaboration of these activities, and his growing recognition of his anger and conflict over continuing to pursue these actions, led him to gradually relinquish them, and improve his relationship with his father.

This allowed us to begin to understand his relationship with his mother, of whom we had heard little. He felt powerful over her in debates and at times reduced her to tears, which increased his contempt for her and her weakness, as well as increasing his guilty feelings. In this context, he recalled being awakened in the late evening by his mother's screaming from her shower. He rushed into her bathroom to find her crying, with blood streaming down her legs. Of significance was A's anger and disappointment that his father was away, and his helpless fear at seeing her bleeding and wounded. He recalled going with his grandmother to the hospital and waiting while the doctors helped his mother, not knowing what was happening. This was the first I had heard of this early trauma in his life. This event was later confirmed by his parents.

This trauma made a profound impression on him, and was reinforced by parental nudity through his latency years. He also slept in the parental bedroom from age 6 through 9, after the birth of his sister. A felt a responsibility for her well-being. She was born prematurely and had monitors attached to her which emitted an alarm if she stopped breathing. He recalled being the first one to hear the alarm, and crying out for his parents to awaken and tend to his sister. This material emerged in the context of his experiencing insomnia, which he associated with his fear and vigilance to be prepared for something bad happening at night (like the father who had to be prepared for the worst with the gun in his car), and not be awakened in panic. His explanation that he had inherited his allergies from his father when his sister was born, was a reflection of his angry identification with his father and his ambivalence toward his sister. I was impressed with A's persistence and determination to understand and master his anxiety and conflicts. I also thought this material reflected his unconscious rage toward his mother for the birth of his sister, and his unconscious death wishes toward his sister. This unresolved aggression and his guilty feelings interdigitated with his severe castration anxiety based on the early trauma of his

bleeding mother who was miscarrying. It had been augmented
by the numerous deaths in his life including the recent trauma
and loss around the death of his maternal grandfather, that had
stirred up all the earlier anxiety.

The continuing work led to A's increasing resistance and fear
of coming to the office. The encouragement of his mother and
our alliance enabled us to explore his fear of feeling better, and
talking more openly of his sexual activities and his "distorted
sexual development." Additionally, he had a "weird" thought
that he wanted to kill me. This I connected with his disappointment that I, like his father, had not protected him from being
yelled at, nor the frightening experience of finding his mother
injured and bleeding. Behind this material, I thought he feared
the closeness and homosexual feelings in our relationship. A wondered about his parents' seeming ease with his sexual behavior.
For example, he recalled an occasion in which his girl friend was
in his room lying on top of him when his father entered the
room. The father said "Hello," and then shut the door with no
mention of his son's actions. Did he not care, or was his father
just "cool" about it? As he explored his feelings about his parents'
nudity and their leniency toward his sexual activity, A's bravado
and unconscious guilty feelings emerged. He stopped his sexual
activity with girls. A remarked that he usually responded to the
girl's desire for sexual activity, and experienced his relationship
with the girl as a "power trip." This was part of his identification
with his father; it held little or no sense of shared intimacy or
mutuality. He began to talk about a girl of whom he thought very
highly, admiring her musical abilities. A was quick to point out
he had never had any sexual contact with her, and that they
shared a close friendship. Confirmation of this "platonic" love
relationship came in the form of an erotic dream involving her
and him. He was surprised by the dream. He did not want to act
on it since he was not sure what effect it would have on their
friendship. This signaled a significant change in his relationships
with girls, his parents, and with his recognition of his guilty fears,
and his emerging oedipal struggles. The exploration of A's sexual
activity and his attitudes pointed out the ongoing pathological

overstimulation that had been an ongoing part of A's life from early childhood. These overstimulating experiences had become interwoven with the early traumatic observation of his bleeding mother and his anger at his helplessness. For A the only adaptive–defensive route was to become omnipotent and powerful; this was the road to control his anxiety and aggression.

DISCUSSION

This material demonstrates the importance of trauma in the adolescent period and its antecedents in early childhood. In the first case, Ms. B's early life was traumatic for her ego development since her mother could not provide the auxiliary ego function to protect her from overwhelming stimulation and frustration that led to the deformation of her ego. B could not develop the capacity to expect that her needs would be met or that she would be comforted. The mother's deafness to her daughter's distress led to a chronic state of distress in B, and mistrust of herself and the people in her life. She constantly feared the loss and rejection of the people in her life. She experienced her father's hostile attitude toward her mother, "momma rat" as a reflection of her own rattiness and unlovability. This was amalgamated with her sexual development. She was not only going to be rejected because of her sexual desires, but because of her anger and envy.

She had difficulty developing a separate autonomous sense of herself. Her only solution was to be "good" in her academic work, and to attach herself to her objects as a way of feeling complete. Ms. B's entry into the adolescent period was fraught with danger because of the shaky foundation of her developing personality. She had a high level of anxiety over object loss and body injury (castration anxiety), with a fear of disorganization and loss of self-control. How could she manage her desires for sexual pleasure in the face of her unacceptable anger at her parents and her envy and greed? The death of her girl friend's father and the threat of dental surgery were the external traumas that she experienced as overwhelming, and that led to her ego regression and the brief psychotic disorganization with which she had first presented. These events touched upon her inner death wishes toward her own father and mother and her sense of herself as castrated. She feared retaliation for her angry wishes and for her desires. These fears were overwhelming in the face of her limited capacity to metabolize and manage her anxiety. Although she made good use of her analytic therapy, it was not possible to repair the ego defect and deformation that made her susceptible to object loss and transient ego disorganization. Was this also a result of a genetic ego defect that mirrored the defect of her toes?

The second patient, A, entered into adolescence with many unresolved conflicts. In his early childhood he had experienced his father's disapproval and temper. A had the sense he could not be like his father because he was bad. The trauma of the visual and auditory experience of his mother's bleeding genitals in his father's absence, without protection, produced a sense of overwhelming castration anxiety. The ongoing parental nudity and body exposure contributed to chronic overstimulation. The child's ego adaptive and defensive struggles led to his developing a grandiose false sense of himself with an emphasis on his needing to be powerful and in control. In spite of his struggles he had anxiety symptoms in the form of phobias and obsessional thoughts.

With his entry into adolescence the increase in his desires was in conflict with his anxiety and fear of his anger at both his parents. This interfered with the usual task of relinquishing his parental objects and developing a growing sense of independence and autonomy. Instead, his defensive omnipotence, which was expressed by his adultlike behavior, covered up severe anxiety and anger, and a pseudo-adult self-image. The earlier disorganizing trauma during the anal and early phallic–oedipal period of his life had never been metabolized. (Of particular note was the traumatic incident of his being awakened at night by the frightened screams of his mother and the bloody sight of her "castration.") The chronic repeated overstimulations of his father's temper outbursts, which aroused castration fears, contributed to his pathology. Interestingly, the miscarriage trauma for the child included the absence of his father, who might have been a source of protection from his fantasies of possessing his mother, and his fantasies of her injury as a consequence of his wish. These experiences had led to phobic and separation anxiety symptoms which then were dealt with by denial and omnipotent defenses. The breakthrough of his symptoms was stimulated not only by puberty and its psychological pressures, but also by the death of his grandfather and his limited adaptive ego capacity. The death of his grandfather touched upon his inner death wishes toward his father. The factor of this boy's more solid relationship with his mother was a significant difference in the two patients and was a critical factor in his not having a psychotic disorganization. A's anger at his mother was more on an oedipal level since he felt betrayed by the birth of his sister when he was 6 years of age.

Both of these patients illustrate the dilemma posed by trauma in the early childhood period which is then interwoven into the personality development with the special sensitivity and vulnerability it imparts in adolescence. The question might be asked whether adolescent breakdown and the emergence of symptoms is inexorable, or does fate play a role in this process? One might imagine that given no external trauma the individual might traverse adolescence unscathed. This, however, does not negate the possibility that the stress of the adolescent struggles may, within the psyche of the traumatically sensitive individual, result in overt psychopathology. There are many variables that come to bear on these questions that require further exploration in order to fully understand these complex issues.

REFERENCES

Breuer, J., & Freud, S. (1893–1895), Studies on Hysteria. *Standard Edition*, 2. London: Hogarth Press, 1955.

Freud, A. (1967), Comments on trauma. In: *Psychic Trauma*, ed. S. Furst. New York: Basic Books, pp. 235–245.

Freud, S. (1920), Beyond the Pleasure Principle. *Standard Edition,* 18:1–64. London: Hogarth Press, 1955.

―――― (1926), Inhibitions, Symptoms and Anxiety. *Standard Edition,* 20:75–175. London: Hogarth Press, 1959.

Furst, S. (1967a), A Survey. In: *Psychic Trauma,* ed. S. Furst. New York: Basic Books, pp. 3–50.

―――― Ed. (1967b), *Psychic Trauma.* New York: Basic Books.

Greenacre, P. (1967), The influence of infantile trauma on genetic patterns. In: *Psychic Trauma,* ed. S. Furst. New York: Basic Books, pp. 108–153.

Rangell, L. (1967), The metapsychology of psychic trauma. In: *Psychic Trauma,* ed. S. Furst. New York: Basic Books, pp. 51–84.

Sandler, J., Dreher, A., & Drews, S. (1991), An approach to conceptual research in psychoanalysis illustrated by a consideration of psychic trauma. *Internat. Rev. Psycho-Anal.,* 18:133–141.

Zetzel, E. (1968), The so-called good hysteric. In: *The Capacity for Emotional Growth.* New York: International Universities Press, 1970, pp. 229–245.

2

Trauma as a Potential Psychic Organizer in Adolescence

PAOLA CARBONE, M.D., AND ELEDA SPANO, M.A., DOTT.PSYCHOL.

Our thesis is that the adolescent, whose identity is incomplete and still dependent on external reality, needs to deal with reality, even if this is harmful and traumatic, and to experience his or her own lacks and needs. To borrow the evocative image proposed by Alléon and Morvan (1996), we might say that the traumatic impact with reality in adolescence could have the developmental function of "un coup de pied au fond de la piscine" (in effect, being pushed into the deep end).

Freud's concept of trauma has assumed many different meanings. In his early works (Breuer and Freud, 1893–1895, pp. 8–11; Freud, 1896), the etiology of neurosis was attributed to traumatic experiences in the past according to a pathogenic model based on physical trauma. The economic factor is already significant and is the common denominator in the evolution of the concept.

The emphasis on trauma as a real event faded gradually over the years. The theory of seduction (Freud, 1896) was abandoned (Freud, 1916, pp. 275–276), and greater weight was given to fantasy and fixation. The term *trauma* (Freud, 1916) designated a second event or intrusion, rather than the infantile experience that was the origin of the fixation. In *Beyond the Pleasure Principle* (Freud, 1920), the concept of trauma was linked to the compulsion to repeat, and indirectly to the death instinct. This theme was reconsidered by Freud in 1938, when he described the positive and negative effects of trauma, as well as the tendency to repetition and repression.

Our definition has its roots in Freud's 1916 view: "Indeed, the term 'traumatic' has no other sense than an economic one. We apply it to an experience which within a short period of time, presents the mind with an increase of stimulus too powerful to be dealt with or worked off in the normal way, and this must result in permanent disturbances of the manner in which the energy operates" (p. 275). This definition saw the light of day during a period when it was already clear to Freud that the cause of neurosis had to be sought in the interaction of pathogenic experiences in childhood, in which lay the origin of the fixation, and the triggering event.

This definition permits us to distinguish trauma (and this is very important clinically) as an acute psychic phenomenon triggered by an external event from the concept of *cumulative trauma*. The concept of cumulative trauma, proposed by Khan (1974), even though it can be linked afterwards to actual pathogenic situations, comes into being stealthily and continuously over time. He says: "One treacherous aspect of cumulative trauma is it operates and builds up silently throughout childhood right up to adolescence" (p. 301), a situation very different from the trauma described by Freud (1916).

The fact that the traumatic experience is characterized by an acute reaction due to a real experience (Freud [1916] specified "within a brief space of time") also justifies another important clinical distinction. Due to the particular situation (time, place, circumstances, etc.) of the trauma, it has a clearly subjective coloring and leaves its mark in the consciousness and memory of the person who experiences it, just like any other sudden change. The patient may not have understood anything of the profound significance of the upset he has suffered, but nevertheless it will be clear immediately that what has been experienced is new and extremely important.

We make these phenomenological distinctions with a view to delimiting the characteristics of the traumatic experience that we have in mind. It is an experience that, given the nature of psychic phenomena, occurs in the subject as an intense, painful, and overwhelming reaction. It can be compared with another psychic phenomenon that was not very extensively studied after Freud, namely the nightmare. And just as with the nightmare, it becomes inevitable that we must try to understand the metapsychological significance of these painful experiences.

Metapsychology immediately brings us face-to-face with problems, since in the development of Freudian thought the significance of a trauma (and the nightmare) is closely bound up with the mechanism of the compulsion to repeat. Therefore, it is also tied to such complex and debated concepts as Nirvana and the death instinct.

This link is formally brought out in Freud's *Moses and Monotheism* (1938). Speaking of the defensive reactions to the traumatic experience, here Freud distinguishes two categories: the reactions of fight and flight; and the particular reactions that seek to make the trauma operate all over again, a living repetition of the forgotten experiences in keeping with the model of the fixation and the compulsion to repeat (p. 74).

The problem is still open and of great clinical importance. Is the trauma, as a particular way of making contact with a painful experience of long standing, lived with a view of transforming the experience by abreaction and/or elaboration of the fantasies connected with it? Or should it be considered part of the compulsion to repeat, and therefore in the service of efforts at mastery?

In proposing a view of trauma as a potential psychic organizer, we place ourselves on the side of authors such as Fairbairn (1952), Balint (1952, 1969), Bowlby (1960), and Winnicott (1965), who emphasized object relationships and shifted from the Freudian one-body psychology to a two-body psychology. These authors identify the origins of pathology in the early and real environmental deficits, with emphasis, from a theoretical as well as a technical point of view, on the patient–therapist relationship.

This choice derives mainly from our clinical experience, and perhaps more to the point, from having worked with *many* adolescents. Working with patients during this developmental stage allows us to observe the interlacing between fantasy and reality, and the external and internal world. The type of adolescents to whom we refer often initiate their call for help by narrating and/ or repeating traumatic experiences.

CASE ILLUSTRATIONS

The two clinical vignettes concern two adolescent females who were treated with psychoanalytic psychotherapy with three sessions per week. They are very different in the gravity of their pathology, but have in common the centrality of the traumatic experience. We chose, in describing the two cases, only that part of the clinical material which seemed most suitable for highlighting the psychopathological and relational meaning of the traumatic experience in adolescence.

CASE 1, IMMACOLATA: TRAUMATIC EXPERIENCES AND A DEMAND FOR HELP[1]

Immacolata began therapy at age 19, pressed by her own need to talk about her problems with somebody. Immacolata's mien at our first encounter immediately put me in contact with her conflicting emotions. She was intelligent and determined, but her face expressed bewilderment, dismay, and confusion.

"I'm Immacolata," she began at the door, and then continued:

I'm epileptic, but have made a real mess. On New Year's Eve I found myself in Vienna with my friends, but didn't want to go to the party with them. I can't bear parties, birthdays, because the day of my birthday is also the anniversary of mother's death, who died giving birth to me and my sister. I, therefore, didn't want to go with them and remained by myself in the hotel room. I switched on the television, but it was all in German. I couldn't understand a thing and was bored. So I went down to the bar. It was practically empty. Everyone had gone to the party. I started drinking vermouth, which I adore because it is sweet,

---

[1] This patient was treated by Dott. Angiolina Di Reto.

even though I knew I shouldn't on account of the epilepsy medication I take. Rather, I think I drank only because I knew I wasn't supposed to. I got drunk. The waiter sat down beside me and we started talking. I took this boy by the hand and led him up to my room and had intercourse with him. It was my first time. Immediately afterwards I got rid of him. "It's a game," I told him as I opened the door, "I don't know who you are and I don't really want to know."

As soon as he had gone I felt really horrible. I felt so bad inside that I went to the window and had a strong urge to put an end to it all. Why should I go on living? There was nothing positive in my life. I'd had a boyfriend whom I thought I was very fond of, but left him for no reason. Now my relations with other boys are nothing but whims. There is no affectionate involvement. My life is marked by the medicine timetable and prohibitions. The neurologist has forbidden everything. I mustn't have intercourse, mustn't stay out late, can't go to the sea because of the waves, can't drive a car, can't go out by myself, and shouldn't even work. In front of the window, all by myself, I suffered like a dog and felt that I had been driven to do something that was wrong on account of the way I did it, not for its own sake. I often do wrong things that make me feel bad. I live out of spite, go against the stream, but this always makes me feel worse. Where could there be a solution? In becoming docile and obliging? But I just can't do that.

I left the window and threw myself on the bed and started crying desperately. I hadn't cried for years, and at the height of my despair I said to myself: either you throw yourself out of that window or you have to find help. It's been three years that I've lived in fear on account of this illness, which came right out of the blue. I go through the treatments without understanding what is happening to me. When I think of that night in Vienna, it seems to me that I lived a tremendous nightmare, but in the end I didn't throw myself out of the window and now I'm here.

Immacolata was orphaned at birth, due to her mother's death in childbirth. She and her twin sister were reared by her paternal grandmother. Her childhood was full of illnesses and disturbances. In elementary school she had scoliosis requiring an orthopedic corset and a program of special gymnastics. She had to wear orthopedic shoes due to a foot defect. Her vitality and, above all, her femininity were curbed almost from the start. Indeed, following these constrictions she decided to wear only slacks in an attempt to hide the corset and the shoes. Frequent illnesses caused her to miss school.

At age 15, she had "nervous gastritis." At that time she met a boy with whom she became involved. Two years later the boy had a serious high-speed car accident and suffered numerous fractures. From that moment on, Immacolata lost interest in him, and left him after a very minor quarrel. She had a profound sense of bitterness without understanding the reasons that led to her rejecting him.

During her last year at school she had her first *grand mal* seizure. Immacolata felt that this illness, which she did not understand, invaded her whole life. Her medication made her feel tired, listless, and discouraged. She decided to interrupt her studies. This was the beginning of the depressive phase that preceded the traumatic experience described, and her decision to commence psychotherapy. During the whole session Immacolata spoke slowly and clearly, and tried to give every detail of the trauma.

The therapist listened in silence, touched by the long and vivid account. The violent emotional reaction seemed out of proportion since more troublesome events in her life (i.e., the recent diagnosis of epilepsy) did not cause such an intense and upsetting reaction.

Immacolata is an adolescent and it is possible to hypothesize that the sexual encounter was based on the need to demonstrate to herself that she was attractive as a woman and defend against her chronic feeling of being defective due to orthopedic and neurologic insults.

However, what struck the therapist most was her story of marked early deprivations (her mother's death), and somatic pathologies. Her story of mute suffering seemed to have found a way to be expressed, at long last, "thanks to" that dreadful night.

CASE 2, ENRICA:
TRAUMATIC EXPERIENCE AND THE PSYCHOTHERAPY PROCESS[2]

Enrica, age 18 years, was referred by a colleague as an emergency because of a sudden decline in her schoolwork a few months

---

[2] This patient was treated by Dott. Eleda Spano.

before her school-leaving exam. She seemed to have lost confidence, was confused and bewildered. Her parents reported that she cried a lot, stayed in her room for days on end, was irritable, especially with her mother, and often highly aggressive.

Almost *en passant,* it was mentioned that possibly she had been raped a few years before, but it was uncertain. I was warned that Enrica had terminated her previous therapy after one session.

From the first encounter Enrica burst into my consulting room and my mind in a manner that I only recognized much later as being clearly traumatic to me. Notwithstanding the appointment made by telephone, she misunderstood the time, and rang the bell frantically while I was with another patient. Since she did not obtain a response, she went downstairs and tackled my concierge in a very aggressive manner, literally bombarding her with personal questions about me. When at last she was seated in front of me, she expressed herself in scornful terms about the setting, which she found less elegant than a colleague's, and my looks. She said that she had not felt like starting therapy with the other doctor because she was too beautiful, since she did not trust women who were beautiful and young. Fortunately, I seemed sufficiently ugly and old, even though I did not have a particularly intelligent air.

The first session brought out, above all, elements of the relationship with her mother, which she described as fused, intrusive, filled with hate and mutual exploitation. She indicated a "mad" mother who drove her mad, and an absent father, "too busy, too intelligent." Not a word was aid about the sexual violence, until she was at the door, when she turned and said: "Ah, doctor, I wanted to tell you that I was raped when I was 15." This was said without any particular inflection or emotion, almost as if she had left a visiting card or shown an identity card. For a long time afterwards she never returned to the subject.

Enrica was the second child, born shortly after her sister to well-off parents who were professionals. They were both of modest origin, but with great social ambitions. For this reason they had always interfered with her friendships and choices. They provided a scale of values and a series of models with which she could not identify and which she despised. For as long as she could remember her parents had been very quarrelsome and violent. The father was continually unfaithful. The mother ventilated and told the girls the crudest details of the parents' sexual life and the betrayals.

Enrica felt trapped by her mother and obliged to think her thoughts. She kept away from her father. She felt bossed by her sister, who drew her into, or excluded her from, her own circle of friends according to the whim of the moment. She was often exposed by her sister to situations in which she was derided or humiliated on account of her peculiarity, which consisted of bizarre behavior.

In the first session her orientation and reality testing were poor. She could not read a watch, and confused the days of the week and the months of the year. Nevertheless, she managed to maintain an apparently functional margin on the basis of an imitative false self and intellectualized defenses. The boundaries between self and object were labile and shifted, just as her projections were intense and continuous.

Even her physical appearance and clothing were out of the ordinary and indefinable. Her delicate, almost Botticellian face, with large sky-blue eyes and a mass of blonde hair (pulled back tightly by a rubber band), were in striking contrast to her body, which was lean, without a bosom, and not really either feminine or masculine. She often wore showy earrings that accentuated the disturbing impression of a head totally separated from the body, which was almost a concrete expression of her practically insoluble dilemma of choosing a sexual identity.

All the boys she met were homosexuals, and she thought of herself as a lesbian. She was looking for a real man who would make her feel like a woman, but every time she found one, she perceived only his brutality and violence. She was disgusted about her parents' sexual intercourse scenes. Her bedroom was near theirs, she heard their noise, and imagined something terrible and violent happening there. The father, in fact, seemed to be very rude toward the mother, and sometimes beat her.

Her relationship with me was always balanced on the razor's edge. Enrica reacted with disdain and belittlement to every attempted interpretation. She tried to seduce me, only to immediately feel herself perilously seduced. She intruded concretely in my life, appeared unexpectedly without an appointment, failed to keep appointments, neither calling nor offering an explanation.

The creation of a therapeutic alliance seemed unattainable. In the transference I was an intensely persecutory, exciting, and ambiguous object like her father, or intrusive and perverse like her mother. She devalued me to the extent to which her need to idealize me made her feel inadequate and impotent. Using the countertransference as a foothold, I sometimes interpreted the violence of her style of relating as an attempt to defend herself against some unmentionable trauma she felt she had suffered, and for which there seemed to be no words. Later, she found the words and told me something that she recalled as a nightmare.

At 15, while on holiday in Sicily with her maternal grandmother (a warm-hearted woman to whom Enrica was strongly attached), she had been courted by some boys. "I was beautiful then. You won't believe that." She hung around with her sister's group and felt small. Probably she had behaved quite intentionally in a provocative manner with the boys, and the reaction of the boys' fiancées was not long in coming. One evening, with the complicity of her sister and some cousins, they seized her, took her to the beach where, while menacing her with sticks, they undressed her and made her climb on a fence to "verify that she was still a virgin." After having insulted her and warned her not to continue with her provocative behavior, they left her for the night without clothes, humiliated and terrorized. She did not remember how she managed to return home, but recalled going to her grandmother to whom she told the event, certain that she would be protected and defended. Grandmother did not believe her, but enjoined her not to tell anybody about it, almost as if she were the guilty party. Then she called her parents to take her back home.

A few sessions later she described the violence of men, which chronologically may have preceded, or caused the above event. She had a crush on the son of a famous judge (Enrica's father was a lawyer), and agreed to accompany him to the family's house in the country. There, instead of the courting she expected, he had brutally given her the choice of anal intercourse or fellatio. She cried while telling this and, between one sob and the next, said: "I didn't even know what it meant." It seems that he eventually sodomized her. On leaving the house, he duly boasted of his prowess to all his waiting friends. Enrica claimed only a vague recollection of it all, but had a very clear image of grazing horses and their heads turning slowly to and fro. As if in a dream, she associated this with her recent passion for riding and the unexplainable fear that horses arouse in her.

The emergence of the two accounts of trauma was possibly the construction of a plausible sequence of events on the basis of elements of reality that are not necessarily factual. For some time, indeed, I, just like her grandmother and parents, thought that these accounts were delusional.

Preceding these revelations, a good object had appeared in the patient's analytical material. This was a governess who sat on her bed in the evening to calm her so she could sleep, had a good odor, and cooked apple tarts for her. In parallel, she began to note with pleasure the high ceilings of my consulting rooms, which she had always derogated, the good scent that met her on arrival, and the old picture in the hall. The account of the sexual trauma emerged in this ambience at the time of her Sicilian grandmother's death, when she was alone in Rome because her sister and parents had gone to the funeral. She didn't want to attend it because she felt too weak to face this loss. She decided instead, despite her parents, to attend her regular sessions.

The account was followed by Enrica's gradual reintegration. She now kept her appointments with greater punctuality and regularity. She resumed washing and generally caring for herself after a long period of almost complete neglect. She even managed to convince her parents to permit her to live in a flat of her own, though in the same building. This made it possible to extract herself from the continual intrusions that living with them inevitably implied. She faced the anxiety caused by this first separation with great courage, conscious of her need for individuation. Almost all the boys who continued to hang around her (often declared homosexuals) were told almost right away that she had been raped. This made it possible for her to justify her disconcerting behavior. After having practically seduced them, she rejected them in a state of terror, shaken by sobs and trembling that she could not control.

She passed her school-leaving examination, then went to the university, where she passed some examinations with fair results. She became more selective in her choice of boyfriends. For some months she succeeded in maintaining a more stable, though still embattled, relationship with a heterosexual male that was based more on tenderness and reciprocity than sexuality. Her social relations improved, and she managed to develop some friendships on her own. Relations with her parents (subject always to the limits imposed by their personal pathologies and their obstinate refusal to be treated) became less violent and more amenable to being viewed in terms of conflict.

DISCUSSION

The different psychopathological characteristics of the two cases (the first in the psychosomatic area, the second in borderline pathology realm) are self-evident, as are also the different functions performed by the traumatic experience.

For Immacolata, accustomed to suffering somatically, it was an occasion for making contact with the existence of psychic pain, the link between her birth and her mother's death. The drama of New Year's Eve culminated in the very significant sequence of a sexual relationship in which Immacolata first invited, and then brusquely rejected, the object. This sequence evokes the symbolic significance of the fort-da game of the wooden reel described by Freud (1920). Immacolata could not get her wooden reel back, whereas the baby observed by Freud could. As we have said, she had left her first boyfriend, apparently without suffering, after he had a car accident while driving recklessly and risking his life. On New Year's Eve, which she associated with her mother's death, she enacted the same sequence with the waiter, repeating the brief contact followed by the irreversible loss of her mother.

Through this dramatization, Immacolata succeeded in passing from the concrete and passive modality of experiencing suffering (we would recall the long sequence of somatic pathologies) to a symbolic modality that enabled her to recognize herself not only as victim, but also as the artificer of her fate.

The part of herself she encountered on that dreadful night certainly overwhelmed her. However, as she commented with a touch of irony during the session, it led her to seek help and not to throw herself out of the window.

The traumatic experience in the second case did not convey any self-reflective elements. Bearing in mind that Enrica's psychic structure was less well-organized than Immacolata's, it would seem that the physical violence had the function of giving shape to, and concretizing, her diffuse and disorganized parts.

In fact, the plot of her account contained and condensed within a single likely event the entire range of archaic fantasies and anxieties that she had previously brought to therapy. Since it was so fragmentary and cryptic it was difficult to offer any interpretation. Her recovered memory of the trauma seems to have enabled her to reestablish a fragile contact with reality. Simultaneously, she could now voice the serious shortcomings of the first object relations that could not be integrated or communicated without provoking in the other object (therapist, parent, boyfriend, girl friends) that selfsame thought blockage, anxiety, and rejection of herself that she had felt from birth. It was not by chance that shortly after sharing the account of the violence with the therapist, she recalled that her mother had once told her that she had wanted to abort her when she first realized she was pregnant. This was based on the idea that her life would be much better without Enrica, and her husband would give her more attention.

It is fairly obvious that the gravity of this patient's condition derived from archaic phases of her mental life, from defects in the narcissistic aspects of her personality. Therapy continued to be very problematic even after the account of the trauma had emerged. The sharing of that data and having accepted it as real, enabled her in some way to historicize herself, to reestablish a link with reality and time, to find a comprehensible cause for, and the origin of, her suffering. This understanding was also more in keeping with her age. It was more efficacious than any other attempt to make her approach the menacing, sadistic, and destructive primal scene, and the disturbing combined figure of her unconscious fantasy. The sexual violence she suffered as a defenseless girl which she had to suppress immediately, due to her family's injunction, provided her with a hook to which she could anchor her sense of fragmentation and confusion. For the therapist it was a thread that could be followed backwards to the long-standing sufferings, and was a key for interpreting the intense, and at times intolerable, countertransference reactions.

The traumatic experience in Immacolata's case introduced the symbolic into a history wholly anchored in the somatic domain. Enrica's trauma offered her a bodily and tangible frame or organizer, somatic violence, for a diffuse identity and fragmented ego. Keeping in mind this relative difference, we shall now try to adumbrate the peculiar characteristics of trauma by extrapolating the common features of the two cases.

TRAUMA AND NIGHTMARE

Both Immacolata and Enrica described the state of consciousness accompanying their trauma by using the metaphor of the nightmare. This analogy, albeit at a different level, was also underscored by Freud (1920). It led him to reflect that just like the compulsion to repeat (likewise linked with trauma), the nightmare and traumatic neuroses constitute a trial for the pleasure principle and the homeostatic function of the psychic apparatus.

On the other hand, in *The Interpretation of Dreams* Freud (1900) stressed that, "the disturbance [of sleep caused by the nightmare] at least serves the new purpose of drawing attention to the modification" (p. 580). In *Beyond the Pleasure Principle* (1920) Freud implied that the task of dreams is not only to protect sleep by satisfying desire: "dreams are here helping to carry out another task . . . These dreams are endeavouring to master the stimulus retrospectively . . . " (p. 32). Analogous to our point of view concerning trauma, a nightmare can therefore be seen not only as an expression of the failure of the biological mechanism, but also as a messenger of necessary awareness. The latter supplants the universal biological need for sleep, and somewhat in the manner of an alarm signal, urges the sleeper to open his eyes to the psychic realities that clamor for urgent recognition.

If it is true that the binding function of dreams partly fails in a nightmare, then it is equally true that an important image has been transferred into consciousness, and that the violence of the emotion, and the brusque awakening characteristic of the nightmare, make it easier to remember the content of the dream. As a result of the violence of the affective component, the trauma and nightmare become firmly impressed upon the memory, and often remain there for years as a point of reference ("a foreign body," as Freud [1916] said). As such, the memory continues to signal the existence of a question to which an answer has to be found.

In our two cases, Immacolata and Enrica attached special importance to the traumatic event. For this reason Immacolata sought analysis, ventilated in the first session, and described the traumatic night. Even though she did not know why, she was aware of its importance. In recording the first session, the therapist took pains to specify how slowly she spoke, and endeavored to recall all the elements needed to decipher it. Enrica seemed to have carried her trauma from door to door for many years like a business card in the hope of finding somebody capable of accepting and understanding her problem.

Trauma and the Environment

This brings us to the second element of the traumatic experience that we should like to highlight, namely, the importance of the environmental response in ensuring that the trauma can preserve its evolutional potential. In elaborating the concept of trauma, Balint (1969) pinpointed pathogenic power, not so much in the violence of the psychic experience as such, but rather in the fact that the other (perhaps the very person who induced it) does not recognize its importance and significance. Greenacre (1971) moved in substantially the same direction when she described the significance assumed by a traumatic event. In the course of treating a young psychotic female, the trauma eventually triggered the healing process after many years of analysis. She said: "I felt that this (the cure) was not due to any analytic interpretations so much as to living through of this past experience in a contact that was maintained on a friendly basis during a period of hospitalization and that counteracted the patient's fear of abandonment" (p. 297).

In our two patients, it seems to us that the traumatic events were lived in a very significant space–time frame. Notwithstanding the discouragement caused by the diagnosis of epilepsy, Immacolata had found the strength and the will to go on holiday with two friends of her own age. Far from home, in a new situation, she had mustered the courage to test herself.

During a vacation away from home, but with her grandmother, Enrica must have hoped likewise, that after the trauma she would find help within the sphere of what she felt was a rather good relationship. But her grandmother did not believe her, and simply threw her back into the claws of a perverse mother and absent father. In this patient the pathogenic significance of the trauma also occurred due to a rejection at that very promising age, adolescence, when it might have been possible, with an empathic containment of the environment, to partially reintegrate the split elements and avoid the development of a psychosis.

TRAUMA AND INTENTIONALITY

The third element that seems to be characteristic of the traumatic experience, and also central for the purposes of our thesis regarding the significance of trauma as a psychic organizer, is its intentionality. Both Immacolata and Enrica clearly played an active part in triggering the events that we call "external," which subsequently made possible, through the trauma, the encounter-clash with the separated and distant fantasy. In a certain sense this intentional aspect makes the trauma resemble action. However, action in the trauma does not substitute for, or cover feelings but, rather, violently promotes a psychic experience.

Therefore, it seems that the external reality of the event was used (obviously at the preconscious level) as a battering ram against the resistance of the ego. It should not simply be seen as part of the dynamics of primary masochism, nor should it be reductively dismissed as a "slave of the demonic." We would rather counterpose the evolutionary significance of the preconscious intentionality of the trauma to the unconscious need that sustained and nourished the compulsion to repeat.

In support of this position we refer to Sophocles' *Oedipus Rex.* That play has provided much food for psychoanalytic thought, and seems to us capable also of shedding light on the significance and the scope of traumatic experiences. There can be no doubt that with the realization that he had killed his father and copulated with his mother, Oedipus experienced a trauma. As an expert writer for the stage, Sophocles handled the succession of events in such a way that the blow strikes Oedipus four-square in the face. This occurs immediately after the reassuring news from Corinth had raised his spirits and distracted him from his obsession. It almost seems as if the script had been supervised by Freud (1916) through the centuries, for he underscores that the traumatic efficacy of the external event derives, among other sources, from its impact on the ego at a moment when its defenses are down.

The impossibility of facing the emotions derived from the discovery is pathognomonic of the traumatic experience. There can be no doubt that Oedipus' reaction to the revelation can be considered clinically traumatic. Yet Sophocles, with diabolic ability, playing on expected news and slips of the tongue from the beginning of the tragedy, makes it seem as if the secret of his origins, which Oedipus is desperately trying to unveil, is already an open secret which is known to all.

At the level of the preconscious, Oedipus already knows what happened, and yet (and it is this aspect that we wish to stress) does not hesitate to face the pain of the trauma and enter into full possession of its truth. When Jocasta, who had long since understood, supplicates him not to question the shepherd "for your own good, and because I love you," Oedipus replies: "Come what may, but I want to know my origin . . . this 'for your own good' has weighed on my mind for too long a time!"

For how long? Is it since the time his parents had decreed his death? Or since the days when he was publicly derided as the son of nobody and "for his own good" his adoptive parents denied it all? Indeed, Oedipus confides that, notwithstanding the loving reassurances of his family, the thought of his origins continued to torment him, "sliding" ever more deeply into his mind. Here we have words that, even at a distance of many centuries, cannot but evoke the ones that Freud (1909) used: "A thing which has not been understood inevitably reappears; like an unlaid ghost, it cannot rest until the mystery has been solved and the spell broken" (p. 122).

Similarly, Guillaumin (1985), and specifically in connection with our theme of adolescent trauma, oversteps the confines of metapsychology. He says, "I would see in certain adolescents' fascination with trauma, as used by the living being, a deep-rooted desire for living, of the possibility of turning to his advantage what in Freudian theory we would define as primary masochism, and thus to propel himself 'voluntarily' beyond his own existence, but with a view to existing" (p. 137).

CONCLUSION

From a traditional point of view, the trauma experienced by our patients can be interpreted as an expression of their structural fragility and of their incapacity to confront the adolescent crisis. It is certainly not by accident that Immacolata and Enrica went through a traumatic experience on the occasion of their first separation from home and in connection with the beginning of their sexual lives. Confronted by the changes brought on by the adolescent process, the trauma acted as a homeostatic device, tending to maintain the preexisting state of things; that is, a relationship with the object dominated by loss in the case of Immacolata, and by intrusion and confusion in the case of Enrica.

While we do consider that the classic interpretation describes the dynamics associated with trauma suitably and appropriately, in our opinion it has the limitation of viewing trauma exclusively as a phenomenon of deficit. It is an expression of the fragility of an ego unable to control instinctual drives and a changing reality. In our work, we wanted to address another, seemingly paradoxical, aspect of the trauma, while emphasizing the organizing significance that this phenomenon can have in adolescence. We obviously do not want to ignore the problematic characteristics of this experience. However, from a clinical point of view, when an adolescent recounts the story of his or her trauma, it seems important to us to consider not only the weakness, but also the strength with which the individual has staged, as in a psychodrama, the problematic nucleus of his or her story.

The analysis of clinical material found in the account of the trauma allowed us to bring out the common characteristics of the cases, as well as the psychopathological complexities of this phenomenon. The trauma, such as the nightmare, which bypasses the defense of sleep as a messenger of necessary awareness, constitutes a way of communicating with the environment. Ultimately, it is an expression of the preconscious intention to face pain and enter into full contact with the past. As we have shown in the discussion of the cases, both adolescents had a long history of silent and unconscious pathology. By triggering the events that produced the trauma, they gave form to a hitherto nameless suffering, and were able to express and confront it.

To offset the tone of a "eulogy to trauma," we should like to redefine such an experience as a particular modality for enhancing consciousness. In some cases this may be the only way in which personalities with particularly rigid or primitive defensive structures can achieve, albeit in appropriate circumstances, and in a manner that is indeed "traumatic," greater contact with split-off parts of themselves, and attempt the adventure of living instead of "existing."

Summary

The word *trauma* usually refers to psychic damage suffered as a result of a negative external act. Based on our clinical experience we hypothesize that psychic trauma is a process through which the adolescent may try to establish inner contact with split-off and isolated parts of himself.

When we consider trauma as a potential developmental process, we clearly distinguish it from those silent pathogenic experiences, such as cumulative trauma. We refer to the classical definition of trauma as (1) a psychic subjective experience; (2) an acute experience; (3) an experience tightly linked to a specific external event.

We have presented two cases of adolescent females. Each young woman requested therapy after sexual trauma. Our intention has been to indicate the factors required to give a maturational meaning to traumatic experience. These are:

1. *Acute occurrence.* As with any sudden change, traumatic experience leaves a mark on awareness and memory, directing the subject's emotional attention to something threatening that needs to be fully understood.

2. *The subject's unconscious or preconscious intention underlying the apparently external event, as revealed by therapeutic working*

through. Many adolescents have already passed through painful experiences without consciously meeting them with their own suffering. In other (paradoxically favorable) circumstances they can succeed in making use of a real external event in order to make a breach in the defensive armor of their ego. Through deeper contact with split-off parts of themselves they may become more aware of their pain and needs, even though in a traumatic way.

3. *The role of the environment.* Trauma sits in an intermediate area between the individual's outer and inner worlds. It therefore helps to recognize the importance of the environment, and particularly of the therapeutic relationship. The move toward awareness represented by the traumatic experience is consequently facilitated.

REFERENCES

Alléon, A. M., & Morvan, O. (1996), Je voulais en finir (I wanted an end). In: *Adolescence et Suicide,* ed. F. Ladame, J. Ottino, & C. Pawlack. Paris: Massons, pp. 114–124.

Balint, M. (1952), *Primary Love and Psychoanalytic Technique.* London: Hogarth Press.

———— (1969), Trauma and object relationship. *Internat. J. Psycho-Anal.,* 50:4–14.

Bowlby, J. (1960), Grief and mourning in infancy and early childhood. *The Psychoanalytic Study of the Child,* 15:9–52. New York: International Universities Press.

Breuer, J., & Freud, S. (1893–1895), Studies on Hysteria. *Standard Edition,* 2. London: Hogarth Press, 1955.

Fairbairn, W. R. D. (1952), *Psychoanalytic Studies of the Personality.* London: Routledge & Kegan Paul.

Freud, S. (1896), The aetiology of hysteria. *Standard Edition,* 3:187–221. London: Hogarth Press, 1962.

———— (1900), The Interpretation of Dreams. *Standard Edition,* 5. London: Hogarth Press, 1953.

———— (1909), A phobia in a five-year-old boy. *Standard Edition,* 10:123–154. London: Hogarth Press, 1955.

———— (1916), Introductory Lectures on Psychoanalysis. *Standard Edition,* 16. London: Hogarth Press, 1961.

————— (1920), Beyond the Pleasure Principle. *Standard Edition*, 18:1–64. London: Hogarth Press, 1955.

————— (1938), Moses and Monotheism. *Standard Edition*, 23:1–137. London: Hogarth Press, 1964.

Greenacre, P. (1971), Infantile trauma and genetic patterns. In: *Emotional Growth*, Vol. 1. New York: International Universities Press.

Guillaumin, J. (1985), Le besoin de traumatisme in adolescence. Une hypotèse psychanalytique sur une dimension cachée de l'instinct de vie (The need for trauma in adolescence. A psychoanalytic hypothesis about a hidden aspect of the life instinct). *Adolescence*, 3:127–139.

Khan, M. M. R. (1974), The concept of cumulative trauma. In: *The Privacy of the Self*. London: Hogarth Press.

Sophocles (c. 450 B.C.), *Oedipus Rex*. Roma: Mondadori, 1963.

Winnicott, D. W. (1965), *The Family and Individual Development*. London: Tavistock.

3

Mourning
in Children and Adolescents

The Analysis of a Bereaved Child and His Reanalysis in Late Adolescence

H. GUNTHER PERDIGAO, M.D.

With the exception of the Frankie case (Bornstein, 1949; Ritvo, 1966), there have been no reports in the psychoanalytic literature of a reanalysis of a young adult who had previously been analyzed as a child. This paper is a report of an analysis of a latency boy following the death of his mother and his subsequent reanalysis as a college student. In the first analysis he was able to partially mourn and resume growth. Under the pressure of adolescent developmental tasks, he regressed and reverted to a withdrawn stance.

LITERATURE REVIEW

The debate over childhood mourning following the death of a parent has yet to be settled. Since 1917, when Freud wrote "Mourning and Melancholia," there has been general agreement that a special psychological process occurs in individuals who experience the loss by death of an emotionally important person. Freud described the mourner as one who is experiencing emotional pain, loss of interest in the outside world, and is incapable of forming new bonds until the work of mourning is completed. While there is a consensus about mourning and failure of normal mourning in adults, there is disagreement as to what occurs in children.

Helene Deutsch, in her 1937 paper, "Absence of Grief," was the first to point out that something different happens in children. Her hypothesis was that the ego of the child is not sufficiently developed to bear the strain of the work of mourning, and that it therefore utilizes some mechanism of narcissistic self-protection to circumvent the process. Deutsch postulated that this mechanism was the result of separation anxiety, and if the ego was too weak to mourn, two responses were possible: first, a massive regression and second, a defensive operation to prevent the ego from being flooded with affect.

Bowlby (1960) took a contrary position by contending that, "The responses to be observed in young children on the loss of the mother figure differ in no material respect from those observed in adults on the loss of a love object" (p. 10). Later, Bowlby (1963) modified his views as a result of criticisms (A. Freud, 1960; Fleming and Altschul, 1963) that he failed to consider the effect of the developmental state of the ego functions on the ability to mourn. Nevertheless, he stated, "The mourning responses . . . seen in . . . early childhood bear many of the features which are the hallmark of pathological mourning in the adult." (p. 521). R. Furman (1964) was also of the opinion that mourning occurs in children. However, certain developmental achievements have to take place. It is necessary to have reached the phallic level of object representation with its inner stability of inner world representation along with the ability to identify and verbalize affect. The majority view, however, is that the process of mourning does not occur in children. Mourning involves the tolerance of powerful affects and repeated demands for reality testing in opposition to strong wishes. It requires the operation of ego functions which are beyond the scope of the child.

Wolfenstein (1966) observed that the internal representation of the lost parent was not decreased in its emotional significance for the child, but rather became invested with an intensified importance. Children denied the finality of the loss, thus avoiding the withdrawal of the emotional investment in the lost parent. She noted, furthermore, "denial of the parent's death coexists with a correct conscious acknowledgement of what has really happened. Yet this superficial deference to facts remains isolated from the persistence on another level of expectation of the parent's return" (pp. 105–106). Freud (1900) had already observed this phenomenon and quoted a 10-year-old boy who remarked following his father's sudden death: "I know father's dead, but what I don't understand is why he doesn't come home for supper" (p. 254). Wolfenstein (1965) described how children in the age range from latency to adolescence cannot tolerate intense distress for long, and quickly bring forward opposite thoughts and feelings. She gives an example of children ages 9 and 10 who cried when they heard the news of Kennedy's assassination, and yet could not understand why their parents refused to go to a movie that evening as previously planned, or were impatient when they could not find their usual programs on TV. In 1969 she stated that the representation of the lost parent continues to be intensely cathected, and there are fantasies of his return. While such expectations persist, there is also acknowledgment that the parent has died. These two mutually exclusive trends of acknowledgment and denial coexist. This is what Freud (1927, 1938, 1940) called the splitting of the ego. In *The Outline* Freud (1940), stated:

[T]he ego often enough finds itself in the position of fending off some demand from the external world which it feels distressing and that this is effected by means of a *disavowal* of the perceptions which bring to knowledge this demand from reality. Disavowals of this kind occur very often . . . and they turn out to be half-measures, incomplete attempts at detachment from reality. The disavowal is always supplemented by an acknowledgement; two contrary and independent attitudes always arise and result in the situation of there being a splitting of the ego [pp. 203–204].

Wolfenstein (1966) commented on the development of hostile feelings toward the surviving parent, which together with the idealization of the one who died, represents an attempt to undo hostile feelings toward the dead parent through displacement onto the survivor. She emphasized that the most intense affect experienced by bereaved children is rage rather than grief. Jacobson (1965) pointed out the coexistence of reunion and restitution fantasies along with the denial of the parent's death. Wolfenstein (1966) views the process of mourning as: "The lost object is thus gradually decathected, by a process of remembering and reality testing, separating memory from hope" (p. 93). She goes on to say a few pages later: "What are the developmental preconditions which make mourning possible? . . . Adolescence has been repeatedly likened to mourning. In adolescence there is normally a protracted and painful decathexis of those who have until then been the major love objects, the parents" (p. 112).

While the primary function of the mourning process is to detach the survivor's memories and hopes from the dead (Freud, 1913), the response of children to the death of an emotionally meaningful person assumes a regular and specific pattern which is very similar to the pathological forms of adults' mourning (i.e., where there is an unconscious yearning for the lost object, an unconscious reproach against the lost object with self-reproach, and lastly denial that the object is permanently lost). The reaction to object loss in children (Miller, 1973) is not to mourn but to avoid the acceptance of the reality and the emotional meaning of the death, and to maintain in some internal form the relationship that has been ended in external reality.

Nagera (1970) emphasized that it is necessary to distinguish in the overt manifestations of the child's reaction to loss those that are a result of the developmental disturbance introduced by the object loss, and those that represent true mourning reaction to that loss. For a child, the death of a parent, in addition to being a traumatic event, constitutes a major developmental interference. There are frequently multiple forms of regression on the side of the drives, a giving up of ego achievements, and development of abnormal behavior. Nagera (1970) raised an important question: How far is it possible to proceed with the slow withdrawal of the cathexis previously attached to the loss object so that freed energies are available for the cathexis of a new object? Complete withdrawal of cathexis from the lost object will leave the child in a developmental vacuum unless a suitable substitute object is readily found. In the latency child, developmental imperatives will tend to keep the parent alive in spite of the ego's knowledge of the reality of the object's death and irretrievable physical disappearance. A child needs an adult to serve as a focus for his emotional reaction, and unlike an adult, he cannot make use of a hiatus in attachment by withdrawing into himself in order to work through the loss.

Fleming and Altschul (Fleming, 1972, 1978; Fleming and Altschul, 1963) approached the problem from another vantage point. They studied a group of adult patients in analysis who had lost a parent during the formative years of childhood many years before their analyses began. At first Fleming did not recognize the significance of object loss on the observable pathology. What was observed was not the initial reaction to the traumatic experience, but the outcome of the patient's effort to adapt to the object deprivation and its effect on subsequent development. The pain was not remembered, but was defended against by repression of affect and denial of the reality of the death. In fantasy, the dead parent was still alive. These patients were extremely difficult to analyze and posed special technical problems. They "were children in adult's clothes." Fleming's studies have helped explain how the mother–child relationship works to facilitate structuring of the regulatory function of the ego and the organization of a self-system which achieves a mature and individuated identity.

Finally, it should be noted that for a child the death of a parent is a sudden impingement of reality on the unprepared ego, which overwhelms the stimulus barrier and the integrative capacity of the organism (Pollock, 1961).

CASE HISTORY

Scott, a 19-year-old college student, returned for a second analysis as a result of difficulties in his first year of college away from home. He had been in analysis for two-and-a-half years between ages 7 and 9. He was brought initially at age 7 by his father because he seemed quiet, withdrawn, and had nightmares. His mother had died two years previously from injuries in a car accident which caused multiple fractures and paraplegia. During the last few months of her life, Scott and his two-year younger brother witnessed her gradual deterioration. The mother would often, while sitting in a wheelchair, reach out and try to hug the boys. But Scott, particularly, would pull away with revulsion and say that he did not want to be touched. During the months prior to her death, she became increasingly depressed.

Following the mother's death, the father had a succession of housekeepers. Scott reacted to the loss of some of the earlier ones, but by the time I started seeing him, he could not remember the name of the current housekeeper.

Approximately one year after his mother's death Scott had an accident in which he fractured his dominant arm requiring hospitalization. A few months later he fractured his arm again. After that he withdrew, was intimidated by his brother, and claimed the teachers disliked him. He withdrew from competitive games, assumed the identity of a cripple, did not make friends any more, and around other boys he felt ashamed and embarrassed. The neighborhood kids taunted and rejected him.

There was little extended family and little contact with grandparents or other kin. Very little was known about the child's developmental history.

COURSE OF TREATMENT

Scott, an attractive child, was frightened, ill at ease, and confused about why he was coming to see me. There was an enormous amount of aggression and reparation in the first few sessions as dinosaurs ripped soldiers apart. The soldiers were then taken to a hospital to be treated. This aggression which was expressed in play, very quickly came into the transference. He began to hide his play from me and it became stereotyped and repetitive. He complained to his father that he was so angry with me, he wanted to run out of the office. Scott felt there was something expected of him, but he did not know what, and that it was frightening and confusing to him. He worried about what I thought of him, and if I had bad thoughts about him. A few days later he stated that I made him think of things he wanted to forget, that I was a mind reader, that I knew thoughts little boys had, and that I was going to be mean to him. He was angry with me because I made him have feelings he never experienced before. The feelings he had in the session were just like the scary dreams in the middle of the night when he used to go to his father's bed. Going to sleep in his father's bed had become a habit justified by the night-time fears.

In the initial months, the analysis seesawed between his intense object hunger and his fears that the relationship would turn out to be sadistic and destructive. He had guilt feelings which manifested themselves in Kafkaesque terms when he fantasied that I would savagely blame him and accuse him of having done bad things, though he himself did not know what they were.

After a few months of analysis, Scott's behavior began to change. As he became less afraid of me, he openly tried to annoy me, bore me, and antagonize me in the hope that I would get rid of him. He also reported dreams, many of which had fire in their manifest content. One day he came in appearing pathetic, crying profusely, saying that everybody was against him, and that he wanted to commit suicide. He told me of a dream in which his street was flooded, which culminated in a statement that if I went by his street, it would be a good thing because I would drown and die. His angry outbursts continued as he told me angrily that I was a creep who bugged him and called him a liar. There were more dreams about fire, and during this stormy period he was miserable. At the same time, he struggled against any kind of positive involvement with me. Trying to break the impasse, I asked if he ever thought about his mother. He said, yes, and calmed down somewhat. I said to him that housekeepers were okay, but it wasn't the same as having a real mama. This was the first time he cried without hostility, acknowledging his immense longing for her and his present loneliness. This open admission of feelings marked a turning point in our relationship. The mood which had been openly adversarial was now collaborative. The nature of the play appeared more typical of a latency child. The aggression was not as raw, and the competitiveness in the games (cards, tic-tac-toe) was no longer a deadly affair. There was a positive employment of controlled aggression in the service of his ambition. Along with this material, he explored his difficulties with his peers. He began to have friends come to the house, and participated in group games during recess. He seemed to be less inhibited and could allow expression of his phallic–oedipal masculinity. He wrestled with his brother and was no longer afraid of him.

This period was shortlived. Suddenly he became totally inhibited. He was terrified of me and thought I blamed him for things he did not do. Finally, he told me in a bland, affectless way that his housekeeper was leaving to return to her hometown. He related how she would take him to the playground, indicating how enjoyable it had been for him to go on outings with her.

From then on, he began to have murderous fantasies about me (i.e., he would become the boss of me and give me a knife and tell me to cut through a high tension wire so that I would be electrocuted, or that he would be powerful and that he would put bad feelings inside of me as I did with him, or that he would make me appear weak and helpless by not paying any attention to me). He assumed the "I don't know" stance so that he would not have to think about upsetting things. I began to wonder if he was about to suffer another loss and learned that the grandparents were about to leave. Just prior to his grandmother's departure, Scott was at his most hostile level, saying that it was not fair that he had to come see me, and that it would be worth breaking an arm to get rid of me, because in the hospital he would not have to put up with me. He became even more furious when I empathized with his bad feelings and speculated how much he would miss his grandmother.

For a while the analysis was very difficult. Scott was inhibited, had little to say, and tried in every way he could to prevent himself from having any kind of emotional involvement with me. I kept interpreting the loss of his grandmother and the maid, but to no avail. Finally, Scott volunteered that his father had a new girl friend and that they were planning to get married soon. He also told me how upset he had been in the gym and that he had an argument with a female swimming teacher. This teacher was reputed to be a very aggressive masculine woman who was very rough with him because he swam so poorly. She suggested that Scott have private swimming lessons with her, but he refused at the last moment and thereafter became phobic about going to school. He fantasied the boys taunting him and teasing him. He recognized that the swimming teacher represented to him one aspect of the future stepmother.

A few days later, Scott arrived in a fury, saying that he had bad feelings but there was no word for them. The more I attempted to elicit his fantasy, the angrier he became. Finally, it turned out that he was angry with his father because he was out so many evenings and was spending less and less time at home. Also, the fiancée spent a good deal of time with his younger brother helping him to read. Scott himself had been slow to learn to read and had considerable difficulties until the third grade. When Scott was with her, he seemed to be very excited and welcomed her signs of affection. Much of the analytic work at this time centered around his ambivalent feelings toward her. He seemed torn: On the one hand he liked her very much, but then he resented the fact that when she was in town he saw very little of his father. Lastly, he started talking about his feelings of loyalty toward his own mother and how he tended to compare the two women. He acknowledged that he had many thoughts, feelings, and imaginary stories about his mother. We talked about her illness in depth. He was a little confused, but stated, with a lot of anger, that his mother had gone to a doctor who did not know what he was doing, and that if she had gone to a good doctor he could have cured her.

In the next few months, Scott was chronically angry with his father. He was now in a different emotional position. Working through the feelings of loss and longing for the mother had substantially reversed the drive regression. He was more openly competitive with the father and ambivalent about his future stepmother. For Mother's Day, Scott wrote his future stepmother a card and addressed it to the greatest mother in the world. He also wrote her a letter saying that he was just waiting for her to come to New Orleans, and that he felt like a rocket at the countdown ready to go off.

In analysis, Scott continued to express his ambivalence. He was guilty about the fantasies he had about the future stepmother, and appeared to be constantly on the defensive and projecting criticism onto me. To relate to her meant betraying and abandoning his mother, and to have erotic feelings about her meant abandoning his father and me.

Just prior to the wedding, the father cleaned house, and took his old wedding pictures and other material pertaining to Scott's mother over to his parents' house. Scott reacted to this with a great deal of anxiety, accusing his father of trying to obliterate and forget his mother, saying that this was not right, and that he could not do this. Scott was not pleased with the father's explanation, and handled the situation by increasing his distance from both his father and the fiancée.

In the weeks prior to the wedding, Scott obsessed endlessly about his fears of the swimming teacher in the fall. He went on saying, "Is she going to expect me to do more than I'm capable of? Last year she had no patience." I commented that maybe he wondered what it was going to be like at home in the coming months. He immediately denied it. He came back to the swimming teacher, and I asked how he could handle the situation in the fall. Though frustrated and obviously anxious about what life with his new stepmother would be like, he did not regress. In his play he became competitive with me. He drew endless mazes which he would trace for an entire session. He bragged that he could follow mazes better than I could, and that he could do it even with his eyes shut. Tracing the mazes was the course of the analysis, and he cockily let me know that he could find his way around the mazes better than I could. He began to challenge me while laughing gleefully, saying that I was not so smart after all, and that he could outwit me any time he wanted.

Another separation from the grandparents changed everything. He presented himself again as helpless and pleaded with me to intercede with his father. He regressed, but the alliance between us was still intact. The analytic work dealt with his feelings of inadequacy. Old themes came up again. He complained that his brother was stealing his friends. He had more difficulty with peers at school during recess. The difference now was that he verbalized these difficulties, and actively tried to understand why this change had occurred.

Then, suddenly Scott became withdrawn and the therapeutic alliance vanished. I received a phone call from his father requesting a joint interview with his new wife so that they could reassess Scott's future. At the joint meeting with the parents, the stepmother seemed to be a chic, pretty, self-centered woman, who was leery of, and hostile toward, me throughout. She made it plain that she objected to the therapy, and that Scott needed to do other things besides come to my office. Her position made Scott's anxiety clear to me and it seemed that she probably had expressed her views to him rather bluntly.

Predictively enough, in the ensuing week, Scott kept complaining about having to come to analysis, and that the other boys would think he was crazy if they found out that he was coming to see a psychiatrist, etc. It seemed that Scott had to carry on an elaborate balancing act. At home he had to minimize his emotional investment in his analysis, and with me he maintained a greater distance so that if he was forced to terminate, the loss would not be so disastrous.

Gradually, he started talking again, and on All Saints Day, he stated that he had been having thoughts about his mother following a visit to the cemetery. He admitted feeling sad about her and talked about his fantasies about her. Then he spoke about his stepmother taking him away from his mother, the stupid doctor who did not cure his mother, and how he planned to take revenge on the doctor. He became pensive and obviously sad. I commented that it was hard to allow feelings like this, and reminded him that last year at this time he had turned these feelings into a fight between us. He stopped, looked up at me, and said, "I guess you're right." Following this session, he went home and asked his stepmother if she minded his coming for analysis. Generally, the trend after that was for him to be much more reflective, teasing me occasionally, but throughout he was able to maintain a working alliance. In a subsequent session, he talked about circus life, about its dangers, and wondered, "Why would a guy want to do this? You could never make friends. You move every week and how do you go to school?" This was followed again by a difficulty with some of his friends and what steps he was taking to correct those difficulties.

Themes of relationships and object loss became more commonplace. He commented that his head says one thing, and that his feelings say something else. His feelings say that if he likes his stepmother, he's forgetting his mother, though he knows that this is not so. He recalled that when he saw his father tear up his mother's driver's license he was furious. Also, Scott told his father that he wanted it clearly understood that his wife would be called "mom" or "mother," whereas his real mother had been called "mommy." He repeatedly expressed feelings that the stepmother was trying to make him forget his mother and how uneasy he felt about this. With a great deal of sadness, he related his recent trip to the cemetery.

Another theme which became more prominent had to do with reflections about his physical abilities. He had felt for a long time that he could not keep up with his peers. In gym he was afraid that his arms were weak, and he felt that he was not like other boys. Not having a mother made him feel different from other children. He felt he had bad luck and wondered if he was weak somehow. He was very uneasy talking about the subject. His ambivalence about the analysis became more intense, many feelings about the housekeepers were revived, especially, he said, "That they were there a month and then left, just as you got to know them." He recalled several housekeepers and he felt they had lied to him. "You barely got to know them, and then they would find an excuse to leave." As it turned out, the motive for talking about the housekeepers was that his grandparents were leaving again as they had done in previous years. He compared his reflective reactions now versus the angry withdrawal in the past. In subsequent sessions, he even allowed himself to cry, and acknowledged how much he was going to miss his grandmother.

Unfortunately, his stepmother began to pressure him more to stop analysis. He became very uncomfortable and told her to stop talking about it. He was also able to notice that he had come in upset and how he was hiding his feelings. He had completely forgotten the conversation with her the night before, and all he knew was how upset and teary he felt during the day. The next association to the denial of his upsetting feelings was to talk about his fractures, of going to the doctors, his X-ray, being taken to the hospital, and how frightening all of those experiences were. He became genuinely reflective and began to understand how he defended himself against frightening feelings, and how these somehow showed up in other places. In the midst of this exploration of feelings and defense, Scott's father called me and asked whether Scott should continue his analysis. He and his wife had been fighting and she resented the money spent on analysis. Scott knew that his father had called me, and after that, he virtually did not say a word for four weeks. A couple of months later he came in tearfully saying that his parents were fighting a lot, and that the stepmother had threatened to leave. She was furious because some mail had come recently addressed to Scott's mother. Scott was visibly shaken about this. In the next several

weeks, there were floods of associations about the different housekeepers and Scott became more disturbed. He frequently asked
me why I was looking at him. He was more suspicious of me, and
very uncomfortable about having anything to do with me. He
had regressed again, and his observing ego which had begun to
develop recently vanished completely. His analysis lasted another
two months, but for practical purposes one might say that it was
over at the time of the parents' last fight. He came in body but
not in spirit. There was no termination. He had virtually shut me
out and was totally unreceptive to any of my comments about the
difficult situation in which he was placed. He was determined to
get rid of me and not to have any emotional exchange with me.

THE SECOND ANALYSIS

Scott returned to analysis following his first year in college. He
had experienced academic and social difficulties. He recognized
that he was not working up to his capacity. After the interruption
of his first analysis, he had managed fairly well for several years.
He related well, had friends, and managed to get teachers to
take a special interest in him. In the first analysis the regression
following the traumatic fractures and his loss of confidence were
sufficiently worked through to allow him to resume growth. He
was able to compete again, to participate in group activities, and
to become actively object seeking. However, the need to punish
himself for his mother's death and the motivation behind his
accident proneness were never analyzed. In his sophomore year
in high school following the death of his maternal grandfather,
he started to feel alienated and withdrawn. His grades dropped
and he cultivated becoming "invisible." By this he meant he
would act very unobtrusively so as to not be noticed by anyone.
Previous positions of leadership in school and church youth
groups gradually began to fade out.

The grandfather's death turned out to be a prelude of progressively more frequent episodes of castigating himself about his
mother's death. While away in his freshman year of college he
again had two "accidental fractures" along with more guilt about

his mother. His self-reproaches and feelings of guilt occupied a large part of this second analysis. His central fantasy was that if he had loved his mother more, he could have averted her death. While expressing these feelings, he stated, "I know this is not logical, but this is the way I feel."

To atone for his insensitivity to his mother's suffering he decided to become a researcher in trauma and find better treatments. He enrolled in premed, but because of his ambivalence he had the most difficulty with the required courses. To make matters worse, his stepmother ridiculed him for wanting to be a researcher. She belittled his ideals and wanted him to make money. Her disapproval added to his conflicts. To study medicine was to be a reparative move to his mother and assuage his guilt for abandoning her for the stepmother. The stepmother wanted him to have feelings, but only those of which she approved, and he was never comfortable with her competitiveness and hostility toward his mother.

In the opening phase, Scott alternated between hostile contemptuous feelings toward me and periods of totally flat affect. He saw me as callous, cocky, and arrogant, and compared me to his college roommate in whom he had confided, only to find out the roommate had made sarcastic remarks about him to the other boys in the college dorm. His first dream in analysis was about his roommate criticizing him.

The sessions were difficult and labored. I would find myself daydreaming and had great difficulty staying with him and following his train of thought. I was uncomfortable with him, and now it was my turn to have feelings of wanting to run out of the room. Finally, I was able to confront Scott with the fact that although he was talking to me, in his mind he was someplace else. He agreed that this was correct and that this was a test to determine my interest and devotion to our therapeutic endeavor. Could he snow me and talk about meaningless material? Would I call his hand on it, or would I just let him go on?

After this initial difficulty, Scott took another tack. He would begin to talk, break off in midsentence and ask me, "Do you know what I mean?" When confronted, his reply was that this was another test. If I was a good doctor, I would know, or at least make the effort to find out what was inside his head. In his first analysis, I was supposed to have been a mind reader. Now he made himself opaque and invisible, and then if I was to stay with him and follow him, I was to anticipate his half-formulated thoughts.

After these opening phase resistances, he began to have feelings that I stared at him contemptuously, and that I was always ready to criticize him. Projecting his criticism onto me had a defensive quality in that he could evade dealing with the past and all of the pain that he felt inside. His self-destructive behavior became clearer to him as he related flunking an exam with a smug, proud smile. When this was pointed out to him he at first dismissed these observations disdainfully, but later acknowledged that he felt guilty if he did well or felt content.

As this defensive denial began to give way, the enormous burden of guilt became apparent. He expressed feelings directly that if he had loved his mother more, or if he had not abandoned her, she would not have died; or if he had done more for her, or conveyed to her that he loved her, she would still be alive today. When he was told by his father that his mother had died, he showed no emotion, and was actually glad to stay home the next day and be able to watch TV. He felt that as punishment he could never be happy. In his words: "I want to stay burdened. I don't want to walk away feeling better. Not to feel burdened is reckless. She is ill right now, and it is like she's still alive in a way. If she was dead, I would not feel burdened. But pretending she's not dead helps me wall off the past and she does not affect everything I do." By admitting her death, feelings of sadness would come into play. "It is an obligation to my mother not to be in the present. It is a betrayal of her to be here interacting with you."

He also accused me of abandoning him as a child with comments such as: I should have done more for him and been more in control, I had been too passive and allowed his stepmother to dictate the terms of the therapy; this could only have happened because seeing him was only a job and that I couldn't possibly have cared for him; had that been the case I would not have abandoned him. Discussing his feelings about me allowed him to explore another set of feelings. He felt that his mother was dead, that she abandoned him, and left him terribly alone. After he was confirmed in church as a teenager, he went to the cemetery with his father and grandfather. He remembered feeling resentful: "She was gone all those years. Why is she coming back now?" This was after his father told him how proud his mother would be of his accomplishments. These two sets of feelings, that she was dead and that she was not dead, coexisted side by side. He felt that he had to have a private relationship with his mother to the exclusion of everyone else. Emotionally, there was confusion about who abandoned whom, as he oscillated back and forth between the two positions. To add to the confusion, his stepmother's incessant demeaning attitude toward him was that what had happened to him was not such a big deal, and that he should quit making such a big fuss over it. He felt everyone had taken his feelings away from him, and that he no choice but to become some sort of ghost. In his words, "I am frustrated that I don't have an identity because the feelings I have I am not allowed to have. How do they expect me to know what I want to do when they want to shut out my past."

Although he never missed a session, once in the office, he stated, "I don't trust you. You only do this because it's your job. I don't want to become personal with you, because then I will be vulnerable and I am going to get hurt. You are the voice of my conscience. You tell me don't forget about the past. Don't forget what you did. You cannot have fun. If I get upset, you will reject me. Your role is to be a negative reminder of my past. How can you have fun? How can you have forgotten that your mother died and suffered a great deal?" Later he added, "I feel like a little kid because I'm afraid to have emotion. I am an emotional icicle now. When I come here I have flashbacks about the past, and I don't want to feel anything."

As the analysis moved to midphase, he began to react explosively to any break in the continuity. Mondays were always difficult. Following vacations he appeared sullen and suspicious. He blasted me for wanting him to spill out his guts while I just sat there. The transference fantasy which finally emerged, was that I was responsible for his life and that if I cared enough for him, I would reach out and save his life. He reached out and was rejected, now it was my turn to reach out to him, and he would reject me over and over. He would make himself unapproachable when he felt bad and dare me to try to bring him out. During one of the interruptions he told me with rageful tears that it was not fair that he was reliving the past through me, and that all his efforts to wall off the past were failing.

Scott felt in a quandary, no longer able to deny his feelings, but still expecting to be criticized for them. When asked how, he replied: "People condemn me if I show feelings in little kinds of ways." When asked how this happened he replied: "When I was a child they would say to me, stop rubbing your eyes; Why aren't you having fun? Why are you so afraid of the swimming teacher?"

He was very conflicted about feelings of closeness. He alternated between being haughty and condescending, intimating that I was a simpleton, or he would be frightened because he would feel that by the end of a session he felt alive, but by the next day he would be a zombie again. When he was particularly contemptuous after a comment of mine, he would roll his eyes and say: "I can talk logically too." He had to remain a zombie because being tuned in would bring on unbearably sad feelings. These feelings invariably related back to his behavior with his mother: "I feel guilty when I respond to people now but didn't do it then. I tell myself you are trying to do something now, why didn't you do it for your mother. Studying is not important in the context of her suffering. To study and shut everything out is being selfish because I should be tending to my mother."

The second analysis, too, was beset with object losses. After the patient was in analysis a few months, his uncle died. At this point all rapport between Scott and myself broke down. He looked at me distrustfully, as if to say that I was responsible for the uncle's death. This was followed by a prolonged siege of silence very reminiscent of his behavior in the first analysis. He finally acknowledged that it had been his feeling that I promised him if he came to see me again there would be no more deaths. Since his first analysis he had experienced several deaths. Besides his mother, a girl cousin died when he was a teenager. Then his paternal grandfather, his uncle, and lastly his stepmother's father died. Scott had actually become close to him, and with his death relived in the analysis many of the anxieties that he had experienced about his mother. Again, he reproached himself for not doing enough for him, and that he in some way felt responsible for the man's death. Scott was also convinced that as a punishment, he would eventually die of paralysis.

Another aspect of Scott's analysis has been an introject which he calls his intermediary mother. He created this construct in grammar school to protect him from abandonment. Later in high school this introject tortured and persecuted him. It prevented him from having relationships with people and getting in touch with his real mother. This was the image of a vengeful, angry mother bent on punishing and hounding him. He struggled with the feeling that if he was successful, he was abandoning his mother, and that only by being a failure could he stay at one with her. He realized that if he did well in two consecutive tests, he would inevitably flunk the next one. He also stated, "All of this persecution, all of this blaming myself for my mother's death, protects the sad little boy. I won't find him, but also, it doesn't let anyone who will hurt him get too close to him."

In the transference his feeling was that there were two of me. The one who was with him in the present was nice, but the one from childhood was mean. After seeing me he had felt good and marveled at the good results that had been achieved. Later, however, he felt that he had been tortured by me for the sake of a good result. He compared it to a medical procedure, "It is going to hurt a lot now, but you are going to be better off when it is over. You were a bad guy then making me think all those bad things."

His relationship with his father was very ambivalent. He felt contemptuous of his father's obsessive character traits and how he would become mechanical when under stress. He recalled how critical he was of his father when the father told the two boys about the mother's death. The father did not know what to say to the boys and began to talk about a fish dying in the sea, trees dying, etc., and Scott thought to himself, why doesn't he get to the point and tell us that mother just died. To Scott, mother had died several months before, and the announcement of her physical death had only been a formality. As he grew older his relationship with his father changed as he arrogantly dismissed his father's statements to him and treated him with utmost contempt. Although he had this contempt for his father he was very subservient to him. The father, a rigid, obsessive rule-bound man, did for his children out of a sense of obligation, but his lack of enthusiasm for the job of fathering was evident. His passivity vis-à-vis his new wife infuriated the patient and only heightened his disdain for his father. Repeatedly during adolescence he tried to reach out to his father, when he had to face another loss, only to be disappointed at his father's lack of responsiveness. The patient knew that his stepmother had pressured his father into making the patient quit analysis, and he was furious at father for not standing up to his wife. It left the patient with a feeling that he really could never count on his father for any kind of support. He despised his father's lack of backbone. These feelings about the father were replayed in the transference in many different ways. Prior to the second analysis he did not openly express his contempt for his father, but once he began treatment again, he related to him in a cocky, callous, and arrogant manner just as he imagined I related to people. Identifying with what he imagined me to be gave him the strength to challenge his father. However, when the patient's school performance was unsatisfactory, his father would then retaliate with contempt and reinforce the sadomasochistic interaction between the two.

The patient got along reasonably well with his stepmother, except on the subject of his mother. One of the stepmother's unconscious demands on him was that there be no past before she came into the picture, that his mother's death was no big deal, and that he should get on with his life and stop this foolishness of castigating himself. He, in return, tormented the stepmother perversely by acting as though his relationship with her had no history and that every day started anew. On the other hand, he was her favorite and very helpful with the children of the second marriage.

Scott's dating was practically nonexistent. His feeling was, "Every time I opened up a little bit with a girl, it was always a letdown." He recognized that if someone expressed fond feelings toward him, he felt a compulsion to break off the relationship and to act in a self-destructive way. With girl friends he has followed the same impersonal pattern by choosing girls who did not demand much of him. Direct questioning about masturbation or sexual activities elicited denials and extreme feelings of discomfort. He gave the impression of being basically asexual, and suffering from massive sexual inhibition. Only after working through his feelings of guilt and loss was he able to cautiously begin dating. Of course, the first girl he chose was from a different cultural background than his, and his parents put enormous pressure on him to stop dating her because she was not marriage material. He could not resist the pressure. Later, when he went out with other girls he felt he had to keep those relationships secret so that his parents would not interfere.

He dropped out of the premed program and chose a social sciences curriculum becoming very involved in campus activities. He became particularly interested in the school's program of help to handicapped students, organizing a set of activities for those students and wheeling several of them around the campus.

He terminated his analysis upon graduation from college knowing that some issues had not been resolved yet. He was still undecided on a career choice and his relationships with girls were still superficial. He wanted to stop to go to work and pay for further therapy himself so he would not be accountable to his stepmother.

DISCUSSION

This case provides us with an opportunity to study several important issues. The precipitating factors which led to reanalysis, the correlation between childhood and adult pathology, the vicissitudes of the unconscious sense of guilt and the resultant self-destructive behavior, and finally the question of mourning in children.

It has been the observation of Fleming (1972, 1975, 1978) that patients who lost a parent in childhood sought help in situations where the pressure of events would result in a separation experience which, if accomplished, would lead to more independence, more reliance on resources within themselves, and more intimate relationships with others. Living in a college dorm away from home brought these stresses together for Scott, resulting in a heightened withdrawal and regression.

With regard to the correlation between childhood and adult pathology, it was a striking experience to witness essentially the same responses to separation and object loss in the 7-year-old and the 20-year-old. Then, and now, the unconscious sense of guilt was acted out, but the 20-year-old could verbalize the transference fantasy and, therefore, make the behavior more accessible. However, the self-destructive acting out continued for a long time.

Freud (1923) was not hopeful regarding the outcome in cases with a deep-seated unconscious sense of guilt. He said: "Nothing can be done against it directly, and nothing indirectly but the slow procedure of unmasking its unconscious repressed roots, and of thus gradually changing it into a *conscious* sense of guilt." But even after that had been accomplished, he felt that "there is often no counteracting force of a similar order of strength which the treatment can oppose to it" (p. 50).

Prior to both analyses the patient injured himself physically, and later he managed to do it with regards to career choice. He dropped out of the premed program because of his conflicts, but was still unable to concentrate because of his daydreaming. He added to his unconscious gratification by getting his family to criticize and ridicule him.

The most central issue raised by Scott's case pertains to the whole question of mourning and its consequences. Freud (1916) in his essay, "On Transience," stated, "Mourning over the loss

of something that we have loved . . . seems so natural to the lay-
man that he regards it as self-evident. But to psychologists, mourning is a great riddle. . . . Why is it that this detachment of libido
from its objects should be so painful a process is a mystery to
us . . . " (p. 306).

In the literature there have been several case reports (Gauthier,
1965; E. Furman, 1974; Lopez and Kliman, 1979; Sekaer, 1986)
of the analysis and facilitation of mourning in young children.
However, there have been no follow-up studies of these children
and the vicissitudes of their development. Once mourning has
occurred, is the process over? Or can there be a regressive revival
of the partially mourned object as a result of further trauma?
Scott's case answers some of these questions since it was clear
that he regressed during adolescence as a result of further object
loss. From the data of his first analysis, it appeared that there was
an emotional acknowledgment of the mother's death. In addition
to her death, the patient suffered repeated object losses (the
housekeepers and later the analyst). His home environment after
the father's remarriage discouraged active mourning and he was
only able to accomplish it because of his treatment.

In her article "On Trauma: When Is the Death of a Parent
Traumatic?" E. Furman (1986) discusses various external factors,
but neglects the aspect of internal trauma when a parricidal fantasy coincides with an external event. Scott's mother died at the
height of his oedipal period. Part of Scott's tenacious sense of
guilt centered around his fantasies of wanting to kill his father.
He atoned for them behaviorally by an abject obedience to his
father's wishes while harboring murderous wishes toward him.
Tom, the younger brother, reacted very differently to the death
of the mother. He became rebellious and engaged in minor delin-
quencies, but did not have a pervasive sense of guilt.

Fleming (1972) commented on the resistances to the development of a therapeutic alliance and unanalyzable transference.
She stated that these patients continued to live out their preloss
relationship with someone who is expected to join in the illusion
that the lost parent is still alive. The first technical test is to understand the patient's need to maintain the internal object world

and how he strives to do it. The patient resists giving any significant meaning to the analyst, and by not acknowledging the reality
of his mother's death, avoids the pain of grief and mourning.
Others have used the technique of making the patient aware of
the analyst's emotional presence by as active a confrontation as
the patient could tolerate. This had to be done repeatedly in
order to be able to tolerate being in the room with the patient.
Fleming's patients were in a state of arrested development. They
had paid a heavy price in terms of sacrificing development of a
mature self and object constancy.

In this case, there was a coexistence of mutually exclusive attitudes about his mother's death. In his paper on fetishism, Freud
(1927) discusses two male patients who lost one of their parents
at ages 2 and 10, respectively. Each patient refused to acknowledge his parent's death, yet neither was psychotic. Freud commented: "Only one current of their mental processes had not
accepted the father's death. There was another which was fully
aware of the fact—the one which was consistent with reality and
stood alongside the one which accorded to the wish" (p. 156).

During his first analysis, the splitting of the ego was harder to
detect because the patient was not able to verbalize his fantasies
about his mother. Also, in adolescence the splitting of the ego
becomes more apparent because there is a greater synthetic function of the ego.

Were the observed phenomena manifestations of grief but not
the systematized work of mourning? Mahler (1961) states:

We know that systematized affective disorders are unknown in childhood. It has been conclusively established that the immature personality
of the child is not capable of producing a state of depression such as is
seen in the adult. The grief as a basic ego reaction does prevail. . . . The
child's grief is remarkably shortlived because its ego cannot sustain itself
without taking prompt defensive actions against the object loss. . . .
Mechanisms other than the bereavement, such as substitution, denial
and repression, soon take over in various combinations. Children recover from transient reactions of mourning accordingly with lesser or
greater scar formation [p. 342].

Mahler's statements coincide very closely with Nagera's statement about the child's inability to tolerate an emotional hiatus and if there is not an object there in reality, it has to be substituted in fantasy.

This case has provided an opportunity to study how reactions to overwhelming trauma are metabolized in the psyche of a child and adolescent and how defensive patterns may have an enduring quality throughout an individual's life without adequate therapy.

CONCLUSION

In this paper we have seen how massive trauma brought about a regression and a developmental arrest. Without analytic treatment this child would have remained severely crippled in his emotional life, and only through intensive analytic work was he able to undo the consequences of his mother's traumatic death. Treatment allowed him to resume growth and cope with the trauma.

As a result, he would have been able to negotiate the maturational task of adolescence, had he not had to cope with more deaths in his family. These reactivated the original trauma and brought about another regression. The final trauma, having to leave home to go to college, taxed his coping abilities to the limit. He could not handle the separation and maintain himself away from home.

In his second analysis the patient was able to verbalize feelings in a way which had not been possible for him when he was a latency child. This provided him with the opportunity to rework the initial trauma and allowed him to resume growth. It has been many years since the termination of his second analysis and he has been able to maintain the gains and continue to grow. He acknowledges that all his conflicts were not completely worked out and is planning one day to return to explore further his anxieties surrounding intimacy. However, he is very satisfied with the results of treatment and feels it changed his life dramatically. Seven years after his termination he sent me a Christmas card entitled "Forget me not" in which he thanked me for allowing him to have a life of his own.

References

Bornstein, B. (1949), The analysis of a phobic child. Some of the problems of theory and technique in child analysis. *The Psychoanalytic Study of the Child*, 3/4:181–226. New York: International Universities Press.

Bowlby, J. (1960), Grief and mourning in infancy and early childhood. *The Psychoanalytic Study of the Child*, 15:9–52. New York: International Universities Press.

———— (1963), Pathological mourning and childhood mourning. *J. Amer. Psychoanal. Assn.*, 11:500–541.

Deutsch, H. (1937), Absence of grief. *Psychoanal. Quart.*, 6:12–22.

Fleming, J. (1972), Early object deprivation and transference phenomena: The working alliance. *Psychoanal. Quart.*, 41:23–49.

———— (1975), Some observations on object constancy in the psychoanalysis of adults. *J. Amer. Psychoanal. Assn.*, 23:743–759.

———— (1978), Early object deprivation and transference phenomena, pre-oedipal object need. Paper presented at a meeting of the New Orleans Psychoanalytic Society.

———— Altschul, S. (1963), Activation of mourning and growth by psychoanalysis. *Internat. J. Psycho-Anal.*, 44:419–431.

Freud, A. (1960), Discussion of Dr. John Bowlby's paper. *The Psychoanalytic Study of the Child*, 7:42–50. New York: International Universities Press.

Freud, S. (1900), The Interpretation of Dreams. *Standard Edition*, 4&5. London: Hogarth Press, 1953.

———— (1913), Totem and Taboo. *Standard Edition*, 13:1–161. London: Hogarth Press, 1955.

———— (1916), On transience. *Standard Edition*, 14:303–307.

———— (1917), Mourning and melancholia. *Standard Edition*, 14:237–258. London: Hogarth Press, 1957.

———— (1923), The Ego and the Id. *Standard Edition*, 19:1–66. London: Hogarth Press, 1961.

———— (1927), Fetishism. *Standard Edition*, 21:147–157. London: Hogarth Press, 1961.

———— (1938), Splitting of the ego in the process of defence. *Standard Edition*, 23:271–278. London: Hogarth Press, 1964.

———— (1940), An outline of psycho-analysis. *Standard Edition*, 23:139–207. London: Hogarth Press, 1964.

Furman, E. (1974), *A Child's Parent Dies*. New Haven, CT: Yale University Press.
—— (1986), On trauma: When is the death of a parent traumatic? *The Psychoanalytic Study of the Child*, 41:209–219. New Haven, CT: Yale University Press.
Furman, R. (1964), Death of a six-year-old's mother during his analysis. *The Psychoanalytic Study of the Child*, 19:377–397. New York: International Universities Press.
Gauthier, Y. (1965), The mourning reaction of a ten and a half year old boy. *The Psychoanalytic Study of the Child*, 20:481–494. New York: International Universities Press.
Jacobson, E. (1965), The return of the lost parent. In: *Drives, Affects and Behavior*, ed. M. Schur. New York: International Universities Press, pp. 193–211.
Lopez, T., & Kliman, G. (1979), Mourning in the analysis of a four year old. *The Psychoanalytic Study of the Child*, 34:235–271. New Haven, CT: Yale University Press.
Mahler, M. (1961), Sadness and grief in infancy and childhood. *The Psychoanalytic Study of the Child*, 16:332–351. New York: International Universities Press.
Miller, J. (1973), Children's reaction to parent's death. *J. Amer. Psychoanal. Assn.*, 19:697–719.
Nagera, H. (1970), Children's reaction to the death of an important person: A developmental approach. *The Psychoanalytic Study of the Child*, 25:360–400. New York: International Universities Press.
Pollock, G. (1961), Mourning and adaptation. *Internat. J. Psycho-Anal.*, 42:341–361.
Ritvo, S. (1966), Correlation of a childhood in adult neurosis. *Internat. J. Psycho-Anal.*, 47:130–131.
Sekaer, C. (1986), On the concept of mourning in childhood: Reactions of a two and a half year old girl to the death of her father. *The Psychoanalytic Study of the Child*, 41:287–314. New Haven, CT: Yale University Press.
Wolfenstein, M. (1965), *Death of a Parent and Death of a President*. Garden City, NY: Doubleday.
—— (1966), How is mourning possible? *The Psychoanalytic Study of the Child*, 21:93–123. New York: International Universities Press.

4

The Psychodrama of Trauma and the Trauma of Psychodrama

MAJA PERRET-CATIPOVIC, M.A. AND FRANÇOIS LADAME, M.D.

Trauma disorganizes and paralyzes the psychic apparatus, but in adolescence it also compromises development. It would be an understatement to say that young people in such situations need immediate treatment. Among the methods available, individual psychoanalytic psychodrama is rarely considered, and yet is often described as an invaluable modality in adolescence, when the illness disrupts the adolescent's development or the functioning of the preconscious.

We shall discuss the psychological effect of trauma on psychic functioning in adolescence from the point of view of fantasied trauma, and the possible therapeutic efficacy of psychodrama on impeded functioning.

PSYCHODRAMA

Psychodrama is a dramatic staging of real or imaginary scenes for a therapeutic goal. The word, derived from the Greek *psyché*

Acknowledgment. The authors would like to thank Max Sugar for his review and helpful suggestions which made this paper so much more readable.

(soul) and *drama* (action, accomplishment), was proposed between the two world wars by Moreno (1946), who is considered to have invented the method. There are numerous forms of psychodrama, each with its specific applications and goals. Among these, psychoanalytic psychodrama is a method used for treating psychic disorders and for investigating various psychopathologies. It is based both on dramatic expression, and on the understanding and psychoanalytic interpretation of the process which underlies the dynamics of the scenes. The use of transference and interpretation distinguish this form of psychodrama from all others. Individual psychoanalytic psychodrama, sometimes called "French psychodrama," is one of a hundred classical psychodrama techniques identified by Ancelin-Schützenberger (1966).

Psychodrama originated in 1923 when Moreno, who was at that time a young medical student and theater lover, created a "spontaneity theater," which he intuitively felt would have therapeutic effects. He drew his inspiration for this technique, which he later called psychodrama, not only from Socrates' maieutics, Aristotle's catharsis, and the beginnings of group psychotherapy, but also from the teachings of Isadora Duncan and Stanislavski, both of whom were past masters in the art of expression. He published his first work on psychodrama in 1946, which he defined as a "science which explores truth by representing it by means of dramatic methods," and suggested using it as a therapeutic method. In the United States, where Moreno had immigrated in 1925, psychodrama developed considerably as a therapeutic method, and remained faithful to the original technique.

Simultaneously, the works of Klein (1932) and others extended the possibility of psychoanalytic treatment to children, for whom verbal association is infrequently available. In a psychoanalytic framework, children's (nondirective) play and other manifestations accompanying it, should be considered as equivalent to free association. From observing children's play, their use of objects and persons, the distribution of roles and the development of scenarios, of movements, sounds, and spontaneous speech, these pioneers were able to assert that a psychoanalyst can have access to the psychic processes of his patient, as well as to their contents, whether these be manifest or latent.

In France, a group of psychoanalysts immediately became interested in these two techniques, and later in their combination. Monod (1947), whose treatment of children with school difficulties was at a therapeutic impasse, and who had been trained by Moreno in the United States before returning to France, started using psychodrama with children in 1946. She integrated a psychoanalytic perspective into this new method and was followed in this approach by other psychoanalysts. They gradually accepted the idea that psychodrama could be used to treat adolescent and adult patients who had difficulty in verbalizing. Lebovici, Diatkine, and Kestemberg (1958) used psychodrama with children, and with young adult schizophrenics and other psychotic adults. Their experience and writings present the basis for psychoanalytic–psychodrama theory and techniques practiced in institutions for children and adolescents in France and, more rarely, in the neighboring countries.

There are two main forms of psychoanalytic psychodrama—individual and group. The latter was developed mainly by Anzieu (1979) and those working with children and younger adolescents. Contrary to individual psychodrama, group psychodrama brings together in the same session six to eight prepubertal patients, preferably of the same sex, with a couple of therapists. Interpretative work focuses on group phenomena more than on individual processes. Kestemberg (1986) clearly established the advantages of individual psychoanalytic psychodrama.

In the United States, psychodrama techniques developed without reference to psychoanalysis. Our impression is that psychodrama in the United States and other English-speaking countries does not currently have a psychoanalytic basis, and is closer to "spontaneity theater," "role-playing," "dramatic expression," and "therapeutic theater" (Corder and Whiteside, 1990; Kipper, 1992).

Most psychodrama techniques recognize the topographic organization of the psychic apparatus and their aim is to bring unconscious contents into consciousness through repetition and discharge. Psychoanalytic psychodrama aims at a reorganization of the patient's defensive organization either when it is deficient, or too expensive from the economic point of view (predominance of so-called psychotic defense mechanisms—splitting, denial, and projection; or neurotic mechanisms subsumed by repression). This means that it is also based on the assumption that there can be mutative repetition only if the "transferential links between the patient, the co-therapists and the play director are illuminated by the patient's past" (Bourgeron, 1984, p. 1449). The therapeutic uses of transference and countertransference are fundamental to this approach in order to understand and interpret during the play and the play itself. This implicitly presupposes that the psychodramatists are experienced psychoanalysts or at least therapists with a past or present personal psychoanalysis.

ARRANGEMENTS

Psychodrama can be practiced in a hospital setting, a day hospital, or an outpatient clinic. Our own experience has been at the adolescent outpatient consultation center in Geneva, which is also a teaching center for physicians and psychologists specializing in psychiatry or psychotherapy. The expense of bringing together experienced psychoanalysts with younger trainees when there is only one patient, is balanced by the great benefit for the training process, at least when the latter is based on a psychodynamic understanding of adolescent psychopathology.

The psychodrama should take place in a room large enough to offer the possibility of creating two distinct areas, one where the play will be staged, and one for the verbal exchanges before and after the scenes. The play area should be spacious enough to allow the simultaneous movement of several actors. There should be no decor and no raised platform—this allows significant elements of the scenes to be evoked and imagined. Entrance into the play area is represented by the simple fact of getting up from one's chair. This area must be organized in such a way that the representation is facilitated by perception.

The usual frequency of the sessions is once a week. Their duration may vary from one team to another, from twenty minutes to an hour, but remain constant for the team. Each session is divided into three phases. In the first phase, the play director and the patient decide upon a scene. In the second, the dramatic play occurs, and the working through of the scene by the play director and the patient occupies the third phase. Several scenes, or several variants of the same scene, may be enacted during a single session. The number of sessions varies depending upon whether a short-term (three to four sessions), or a long-term treatment (up to one year or more) intervention is planned.

The rule of free association is replaced here by that of staging and role-play. The patient is asked to propose a theme, stage it, assign the roles to the cotherapists and to himself, and then to play the scene. The physical involvement of therapists and patient invalidates the rule of abstinence, but reintroduces it under the imperative form of "pretending."

The direction of the session is entrusted to a single therapist, called the play director. For a given patient, the play director is always the same psychoanalyst. He has a special position since he is both inside and outside the play, involved in working it through with the patient, as well as interpreting it. Due to this position, the play director is the major object of the transferences. For this reason, he is the one who interprets the play, and links the elements from the past and present. These are understood in the light of the transference to him and the cotherapists. Sometimes, a brief comment on something that happened in a play is sufficient to echo the interpretation already highlighted by the play itself.

The cotherapists always participate actively, either in a role or, if they are not acting, in an "audience" function. The part played by the cotherapists has an interpretative function, for it is always based on a procedure whose purpose is to encourage the illumination of the patient's psychic functioning. The cotherapists' role

can be assigned by the patient or by the play director, but cotherapists who have not been chosen by the patient can also decide to
intervene at some time during the play. In the play they may
represent a range of psychic functions: auxiliary or alter ego, id,
or superego. The purpose is to foster the expression of the dynamics of the psychic conflict, and to stage in the same scene the
conflictual aspects in the mind that the patient's pathological
structural organization maintains separately.

INDICATIONS

In our clinic, individual psychoanalytic psychodrama is considered not only as a form of therapy, but also as an instrument to
help all colleagues in assessing or treating adolescent patients.
During the assessment period, psychodrama can be very helpful
with adolescent patients who are either very inhibited or unable
to verbalize their suffering. It can also be useful when there is an
impasse in an ongoing psychotherapy (see case illustrations below). In the latter situation our original way of working is to invite
the psychotherapist to take part in the psychodrama, but strictly
as a spectator. This enables him to use the content of the psychodrama sessions in order to resume progress in individual psychotherapy.

Indications for psychodrama are linked to the particular mental functioning of the patient and not to the diagnosis. The primary indications for individual psychoanalytic psychodrama are
the disruptions in the functioning of the preconscious. We use
this concept, which refers to the first description by Freud (1900)
of the topographic organization of the psychic apparatus,[1] in order to pinpoint the importance of that specific agency in the
transformation of thing presentations into word presentations or,

---

[1] In our view of psychoanalysis there is no incompatibility between the two descriptions
of the topographic organization. Like many French-speaking psychoanalysts, we see them
as complementary.

to put it differently, in the passage from the visual to the verbal. The patients we have in mind are characterized by their poor capacity to rely on the preconscious activity (very similar to what Bion [1962] described as the contact barrier) to ensure fluid exchanges between unconscious and conscious processes. These patients' preconscious is either too airtight or too porous. In the first instance, it presents communication between unconscious and conscious, as well as the necessary feeding of the secondary processes by the primary ones. This leads to an impoverishment of thought. In the second instance, the capacity for repression is so fragile that the patients are constantly at risk of being overwhelmed by unconscious fantasies which cannot be repressed. Over time we can observe the very serious clinical pictures Kestemberg (1986) described as "phobia of mental functioning." In trauma too, there is an overwhelming of the conscious by the unconscious, and normal preconscious activity is switched off. Therefore, it is evident that any situation linked to trauma may be an indication for psychodrama.

TRAUMA

In Freud's (1920) economic conception of trauma, it is considered as a "breach in the protective shield." The ego is overwhelmed by an excessive flux of energy, which forces the psychic apparatus to bind these large quantities of excitation in order to master them.

As far as psychic functioning is concerned, we can consider that the disorganizing effect of the overpowered ego causes a sort of *topographical collapse*, which crushes and compresses the preconscious. Hence, the barrier between the unconscious and the conscious is no longer efficient, while at the same time internal reality is confused with external reality. The stimulus barrier (Freud, 1895) no longer delimits a space in which sensory impressions and emotions may lead to ideation, where perceptions may become representations, and where affects may be linked to the latter. Instead of being inscribed within four dimensions (outer and inner world of objects and self), psychic functioning is reduced to two dimensions in a surface-to-surface relationship (Meltzer, Bremner, Hoxter, Weddel, and Wittenberg, 1975).

If we accept Meltzer et al.'s (1975) conceptualization, the effect of a trauma could be conceived as a "dismantling of the self," with the protective shield breached and the ego overpowered. Experience is no longer contained, and instead is reduced to the status of events which cannot be dreamed, thought, or transformed, and which cannot, therefore, be discharged in order to free the psyche from these excessive quantities of excitation. The destruction of the contact barrier goes together with what Bion (1962) has called the reversal of alpha function: "even if a personality does not have at its disposal an apparatus which would allow it to 'think' thoughts, it does have the possibility of ridding the psyche of thoughts, just as it gets rid of an influx of excitations: the method used is the reversal of alpha function" (p. 101). Now this reversal attacks the link between thought and its instinctual source, devitalizes thought, and "thingifies" it. The semipermeable stimulus barrier is replaced then by a screen composed of a conglomeration of bizarre objects which paralyzes thought and confines it in a *claustrum*.

In such conditions, provoking a traumatic excitation of this envelope can be considered as an attempt to reactivate cathectic energy, thereby releasing possible countercathexes. Thus, at birth, which for a long time was described from a traumatic point of view only, Meltzer (1985) adds the aspect of discovery, of the awakening of emotions. Paradoxically, the traumatic breaching of a screen of bizarre objects can result in the closure of the gap whereby the inside communicates with the outside, and the reconstruction of a psychic envelope under the cover of the opening caused by the trauma.

"It hurts less to be in pain," is a statement often uttered by patients whom we are trying to help to understand the meaning of their self-inflicted mutilations, suicide attempts, and self-destructive tendencies. They seek all sorts of sensations in an inept or even dangerous way, because their sensory impressions cannot be translated into thought. Indeed, even the representations linked to the trauma are experienced as internal "foreign bodies," and as such are a source of excitation.

After trauma it is quite common to observe inhibition due to the massive countercathexes, or even psychic numbing. Treatment, which is an absolute necessity, is often difficult. Communication may be impossible in cases where the inhibition is too massive. It also may be sterile when, for example, the discussion bears upon the presentations of the trauma, without any connection with the affects. The main difficulty lies in the absence of a space in which the contents can be worked through. It is in such cases that an individual analytic psychodrama is indicated. But can one treat problems linked to traumas by psychodrama? Is it not traumatizing to enact a traumatic scene? Is psychodrama not traumatic in itself? If a trauma is a breach made by perception in the representional world, is it reasonable to add a surplus of perception? How should it be played? What interpretation should one give to prevent the perceptions from being traumatic and disruptive? We propose to examine these questions via two clinical situations.

CASE ILLUSTRATIONS

CASE 1: PSYCHODRAMA OF THE TRAUMA

Vera, who is now 18, suffered from a head injury in a car accident three years earlier, without any other serious physical consequences. After a month in hospital in the neurological department, where she had various examinations, Vera refused to leave the hospital. She suddenly had symptoms of extreme anxiety and suicidal ideas, without a particular discernible stimulus. This made it necessary to transfer her to the psychiatric department.

At the beginning of treatment her therapist often had the impression of being a mechanical respirator whose presence was necessary for survival, but not for a full life, let alone psychic life. A year after the beginning of psychotherapy, Vera repeatedly said, "Nothing" . . . "I don't know" . . . "I don't remember" . . . "it doesn't matter. . . . " But she came to her therapy sessions regularly, and would have admitted herself to hospital as an emergency if her appointment ever had to be changed. The therapist and the patient were deadlocked, tied to the reality of the accident, which seemed to be the etiological basis of her condition, and which, despite all attempts, could not be worked through. The most Vera would say was: "perhaps . . . I don't remember. . . . " As a last resource, her therapist suggested a few psychodrama sessions.

Another trauma rapidly arose. Vera said straight away, "It's because of the accident that nothing's right any more . . . everything was fine before." The play director suggested staging the accident. When the cotherapists began to act like parents who were crazy with grief, Vera surprised herself and us by a first, "NO! It wasn't like that." The psychodrama acted in this situation like the kiss of a Prince Charming and drew the patient out of her state of psychic numbness. The repetition of the traumatic scene in a play context released the countercathexes and enabled other links to surface. By stating her own objection of, "No, it wasn't like that," she gave a sign of a sudden psychic reawakening, and of a redifferentiation between herself and the others.

Although these psychodrama sessions did not solve Vera's problems, they enabled her to retrieve the ability to think. The working through we did together in the two years of psychotherapy following the psychodrama sessions mainly concerned the other trauma which had been hidden behind the screen trauma, and was revealed by the psychodrama. Until then Vera had not been able to think about the rather strange conditions in which the accident had happened. Her father had been driving the car in which she and her mother were passengers. They were going to the next town where her father was to choose a first pair of earrings for Vera, who had just had her ears pierced. The symbolism of the situation escaped no one, not even Vera, who remembered having had a sense of foreboding on seeing her mother's melancholic face. She thought to herself, "She looks as if she'd rather I died." The accident happened a few kilometers from there, and she was the only one seriously injured.

Her participation in psychodrama was brief (three sessions), intense, and fruitful. Two years after recourse to psychodrama, her individual psychoanalytic psychotherapy is progressing well, enriched by the material provided by this brief experience. She is still "remembering, repeating, working through" the unknowable trauma that was hidden behind a "screen trauma."

The paralysis of the psychic apparatus was caused by this "too much." It was too much that reality had confirmed her worst fantasies. This collusion between an event and the fantasies "de-transitionalizes" reality, and the possibility of working through both the event and the fantasy necessitates the recreation of an intermediate zone of experience. Within this zone, the fact that the play is not *reality*, is as important as the fact that it is just this, in *the reality of the play*. The reality of the play concerns both the event and the fantasy, which is then reintroduced and reexperienced in psychic life.

CASE 2: TRAUMA OF THE PSYCHODRAMA

In this second situation, the brief recourse to individual psychoanalytic psychodrama released inhibition. Melinda, 16 years old, suffered from an inability to express herself, although she never stopped talking. Her intellectual functioning was intact, but her psychosexual development had been at a standstill since the beginning of her adolescence. When she was between 10 and 11 years old, her mother became pregnant and delivered for the third time. Melinda, the oldest of the three, proudly slipped into the role of mistress of the house, foolishly rivaling her mother. "Taking advantage" of mother's frequent indispositions, she became exceedingly kind, took charge of the household, cooked tempting meals, and even put on weight. After the birth of the new baby, her mother suffered a very serious postpartum depression, and naturally it was Melinda who looked after her little brother. When the latter learned to speak a year later, he called Melinda, "Mommy." Although everyone found the situation delightful, it was in fact a veritable psychic trauma. Her father's child calling her "mommy" was a particularly threatening stimulus, *after puberty,* to the oedipal conflict. She had struggled against that as a child when she was still protected from the possible realization of her incestuous and matricidal desires by the helplessness of childhood.

At the age of 12, Melinda found herself overwhelmed by anxiety. Unable to reorganize herself sufficiently to continue her development, or to regress, since this was also experienced as a source of anxiety, she became fixed in a state described by Laufer and Laufer (1984) as a developmental deadlock. Her suffering was authentic, but she could never make room for it in a relationship and, although she could recount it, she could not feel it. Her affects could find neither a surface on which to attach themselves, nor a space in which they could be felt. Affects were discharged, words "thingified," and talk was abundant, but lifeless. Melinda suffered from this state and made her therapist suffer with her in the psychotherapy sessions. It was at this juncture, when the treatment looked as if it were going to fail owing to a lack of therapeutic involvement, that we decided to suggest a few psychodrama sessions, while continuing the individual psychotherapy.

In the first psychodrama session, Melinda proposed a scene inspired from daily experience. Her schoolfriends were in the habit of playing together, but never invited her to play with them. She explained that she wished to understand, through this scene, why these young people were so disagreeable. In the staging of the scene, Melinda quickly created a state of total confusion and the cotherapists had great difficulty in remembering which roles they had been given (friend or foe, girl or boy). Melinda was jubilant and walked about easily, reprimanding the cotherapists. Then, gradually, couples formed and made allusions to the primal scene from which she was excluded. Melinda was left alone, and protested loudly (but without showing any anger). At this point, one of the cotherapists collapsed—*as if she were dead.* Melinda became white-faced, and, in a heavy silence, interrupted the scene.

This scene was indubitably traumatic since the *perception* of the representation of a traumatic fantasy had badly damaged the organization of Melinda's defense system. She, who defended herself by a shield of words, evasiveness, and even denial, had let herself be *surprised and penetrated* by traumatic representations which left her speechless. This, then, constituted a new breach in her defense system, whose psychic container had exploded, but which itself *remained contained* within the potential reorganizing space of the psychodrama.

Organizing trauma? Was it necessary to overwhelm the patient by providing her with the perception of one of her worst fantasies? The effect of this trauma was to demobilize the countercathexes, while simultaneously providing the container where scattered elements could be reassembled, represented, linked together, dreamed and thought, with the help of others. The scene forced the patient to perceive the undeniable which had been denied. The recognition of this fantasy which, represented in the space of the psychodrama, coming neither from without nor from within, enabled Melinda to make a first introjective movement in her own psychic productions. The effect of this was spectacular, and this scene marked the resumption of her treatment and development.

DISCUSSION

Of course, one should not expect miracles when trying to traumatize those who are traumatized. If, in the individual psychoanalytic psychodrama we practice at the adolescent psychiatric consultation center in Geneva, we sometimes introduce scenes as intense as those described above, it is also because we have the guarantee of a "triple psychic containment": the patient's, the therapist's, and that of the psychodrama (Perret-Catipovic, 1995).

Indeed, in our procedure, individual psychoanalytic psychotherapy and psychodrama are not mutually exclusive. On the contrary, we believe that patients who are given the opportunity to take part in psychodrama must continue their individual psychoanalytic psychotherapy simultaneously. If psychodramatists sometimes choose to surprise and overwhelm their patients in order to get through to them, it is because they know that before the next psychodrama session (these are held once a week), individual sessions will provide the patient with the possibility of "metabolizing" the residual excesses with his therapist who is present at the psychodrama, but who does not participate actively. Thus, the psychodrama is considered as a potential container of what may spill over from the framework of individual treatment if the countercathexes are no longer functional. At the same time, individual psychotherapy provides a container for everything that was awakened in and by the psychodrama before having the opportunity to work this through. In other words, a safe "holding environment" (Winnicott, 1965) is provided, and therapeutic support or interpretation is available on a regular basis in our setting.

This particular setting provides us with the opportunity to make interpretations in the play, which can be particularly incisive at certain moments, and which would be inappropriate and premature were it not possible to work them through again and again within the framework of individual psychotherapy. However, if some psychodrama settings lead to extremely intense scenes, this is far from being the rule. Sometimes the mobilizing potential of psychodrama, with the involvement of the body, combined with seeing and hearing, is sufficient to catalyze and rekindle a stricken affective process. This material can, after a very brief use of psychodrama, be later worked through in individual psychotherapy.

CONCLUSION

Individual psychoanalytic psychodrama is an extremely useful therapeutic instrument in psychopathological situations in adolescence characterized by inhibition, avoidance, and by apparent confusion of the limits between internal and external reality. Insofar as these signs are present in traumatic states, they are indications for the use of psychodrama, particularly if they are considered as internal trauma, whatever the importance of the external events. Sometimes psychodrama techniques provide the possibility of reviving blocked mental activity more efficiently than individual psychotherapy, and of giving renewed depth to a psychic representation.

In other situations, the traumatic effect is to be sought in the play acted out in the psychodrama. The excitation aroused overflows and puts the defensive apparatus (which has become impermeable due to massive countercathexes) out of action, thus paralyzing all individual psychotherapeutic work. However, in the light of our experience, we are convinced that the capacity for containment provided by our psychodrama setting makes it possible to overcome impasses, and provides a true therapeutic stimulus to these apparently traumatic scenes.

REFERENCES

Ancelin-Schützenberger, A. (1966), *Précis de psychodrame*, 2nd ed. (Concise guide to psychodrama). Paris: Editions Universitaires.

Anzieu, D. (1979), *Psychodrame analytique chez l'enfant et l'adolescent* (Psychoanalytic psychodrama with children and adolescents). Paris: Presses Universitaires de France.

Bion, W. R. (1962), *Learning from Experience*. New York: Basic Books.

Bourgeron, J.-P. (1984), Névrose, psychose et psychodrame (Neurosis, psychosis and psychodrama). *Rev. Franç. Psychanal.*, 48:1445–1452.

Corder, B. F., & Whiteside, R. (1990), Structured role assignment and other techniques for facilitating process in adolescent psychotherapy groups. *Adolescence*, 25:343–357.

Freud, S. (1895), Project for a scientific psychology. *Standard Edition*, 1:281–397. London: Hogarth Press, 1966.

—— (1900), The Interpretation of Dreams. *Standard Edition*, 4&5. London: Hogarth Press, 1953.

—— (1920), Beyond the pleasure principle. *Standard Edition*, 18:1–64. London: Hogarth Press, 1955.

Kestemberg, E. (1986), Quelques notes sur la "phobie du fonctionnement mental" (Some notes on the "fear of mental functioning"). *Rev. Franç. Psychanal.*, 50:1339–1344.

Kipper, D. A. (1992), Psychodrama: Group psychotherapy through role playing. *Internat. J. Group Psychother.*, 42:495–521.

Klein, M. (1932), The psycho-analytic play technique: Its history and significance. In: *The Writings*, Vol. 2. London: Hogarth Press, 1955, pp. 122–140.

Laufer, M., & Laufer, E. (1984), *Adolescence and Developmental Breakdown, A Psychoanalytic View.* New Haven, CT: Yale University Press.

Lebovici, S., Diatkine, R., & Kestemberg, E. (1958), Bilan de dix ans de thérapeutique par le psychodrame chez l'enfant et l'adolescent (A summing up of ten years of therapy using psychodrama with children and adolescents). *Psychiatr. Enf.*, 1:63–179.

Meltzer, D. (1985), L'objet esthétique (The aesthetic object). *Rev. Franç. Psychanal.*, 49:1385–1390.

——— Bremner, J., Hoxter, S., Weddel, D., & Wittenberg, I. (1975), *Explorations in Autism.* London: Clunie Press.

Monod, M. (1947), Première expérience française sur le psychodrame (The first French experience with psychodrama). *Sauvegarde*, 2:50–55.

Moreno, J. L. (1946), *Psychodrama*, Vol. I. New York: Beacon House.

Perret-Catipovic, M. (1995), Quand les mots ne parlent plus: Le recours au psychodrame dans une psychothérapie individuelle (When words have no meaning: Recourse to psychodrama in an individual therapy). *Adolescence* (Paris), 13:143–158.

Winnicott, D. W. (1965), *The Maturational Processes and the Facilitating Environment.* New York: International Universities Press.

Part II

The Trauma of Physical and Psychosomatic Illness

5

The Separation–Individuation Process in Adolescents with Chronic Physical Illness

MAGDA LIAKOPOULOU, M.D.

It is estimated that 5 to 10 percent of school-age children suffer from chronic physical illness (Rutter, Tizard, and Whitmore, 1970). The child or adolescent with chronic illness has to adapt to the characteristics and requirements of his or her illness and emotional developmental stage. Development and chronic illness affect each other reciprocally. Younger children seem to be affected in their academic development (Rovet, Ehrlich, and Hope, 1987), while older children and adolescents have problems in social adjustment (Ungerer, Horgan, Chaitow, and Champion, 1988).

Factors such as temperament and defensive style of the child or adolescent, personality of the parents, marital and family functioning, and socioeconomic status, contribute to the adjustment of the child or adolescent with chronic illness (Eiser, 1990). It is interesting that there are more reports from parents indicating maladjustment of children or adolescents with chronic illness than from teachers, physicians, or data from objective measures (Kashani, Koenig, Shepperd, Whilfley, and Morris, 1988). This is probably related to the difficulties in the child–parent interactions.

This chapter focuses on separation-individuation in adolescents with chronic physical illness. The concept of separation-individuation, which clinically has proven to be very useful, was described by Mahler (1968), who based her formulation on her study of severely ill infants and toddlers. In concept, the separation–individuation process extends from approximately 5 to 36 months, during which the infant separates from mother and takes on its individual characteristics. Mahler (1968) wrote that before the process starts a phase of "normal autism" occurs (0 to 2 months) followed by a phase of "normal symbiosis" (2 to 5 months). The separation–individuation phase was divided into four subphases: differentiation, practicing, rapprochement, and moving toward object constancy (Mahler, 1972).

The rapprochement subphase is very significant clinically. During this period, the infant develops an increased awareness of the mother's whereabouts and insists that mother participate in every new experience because he now fears that the world is not "his oyster." Some mothers cannot accept the child's demands. At 18 to 20 months of age the rapprochement crisis occurs during which fear of object loss is experienced and is related to approval or disapproval by the parent (Mahler, Pine, and Bergman, 1975). Splitting mechanisms become evident at this time.

The persistence of the rapprochement crisis indicates premature internalization of conflicts. In some cases this struggle is so draining that not much libido or neutralized aggression is left for other evolving functions of the ego. This difficulty will make its presence known during adolescence.

In the course of adolescence, a series of regressions and progressions of drive and ego take place (Blos, 1967). In order to disengage from archaic internal objects the adolescent ego has to come in contact with them. Through these processes, the second individuation phase of the life-cycle is achieved. During this period, strong sexual and aggressive impulses emerge which are better organized than those of childhood. In early adolescence, a need for distance from the parents is present because of these impulses. This is the first period of the separation process from parents. In late adolescence, the continuation and completion of this process is generally expected, but to a variable degree, depending on the culture. Also, a considerable transformation of values occurs in late adolescence which results from the attenuation of parental influence and increased influence of peers and adults outside the family. Isay (1977) follows Blos (1967) and Erikson (1950) in noting that the final goal of the completion of adolescence should be the attainment of a firm vocational and sexual orientation.

Sometimes adolescents form unwise relationships, which are destructive. Even these relationships contribute to the goal of expanding the capacities of the ego for control and organization of new reality situations. The needed psychological distance from the parents also contributes to the attainment of this goal. Of course, not all adolescents form destructive relationships. The adequate resolution of preoedipal issues pertinent to the separation–individuation process is needed before the attainment of goals of firm sexual and vocational orientation can occur (Blos, 1967). Otherwise, an incapacitating anxiety comes to the fore and interferes with attaining this goal.

ADOLESCENCE AND CHRONIC ILLNESS

Chronic physical illness complicates the adolescent's separation–individuation process. The difficulties caused by the illness as well as the interaction between the illness on the one hand, and the process of adolescence, parents, social class and culture on the other hand, will be illustrated through the examples of adolescents with diabetes and other endocrine illnesses.

The normative upsurge of aggressive and sexual impulses of adolescence, which occurs simultaneously with the individuation process, obviously affects the course of the chronic illness. This was demonstrated in a study of diabetes in which youngsters, whose illness started in adolescence, had a more unstable course over a four-year follow-up than those whose illness started at a younger age (Jacobson, Hauser, Lavori, Wolfsdorf, Herskowitz, Millet, Bliss, and Gelfand, 1990). Obviously the need to separate from parents and have one's own circle of peers is affected by the illness.

NARCISSISTIC INSULT

Another dimension worth mentioning is the narcissistic trauma created by chronic illness with which the adolescent is continuously confronted. Consequences of this trauma are an alteration of the self-image representation (in fact, a defective body image is formed); withdrawal of narcissistic libido from the self; lowering of self-esteem (Liakopoulou, 1994); and a state of resignation (Spirito, Stark, Gil, and Tyc, 1995). These are features of a depressive reaction. This reaction goes along with the lack of friendships, dates, and popularity among peers about which these adolescents complain (Capelli, McGrath, Heck, McDonald, Feldman, and Rowe, 1989; Spirito et al., 1995). A late adolescent girl with adrenal hyperplasia put it this way: "I withdrew from contact with people because of my problem." It is too painful to be different from the others (Moran, 1984).

PATHOLOGICAL DEFENSES

The lack of friends does not facilitate either the separation or the individuation process. This means that new identifications do not occur, self and object representations are not altered (Miller, 1973), and restructuring of the internal world (modifications of the superego and ego ideal) does not take place to the extent that it should. The difficulty in separation is also exemplified by the fact that some late adolescents have difficulty in making the transition from the pediatric clinic to the adult clinic for their medical follow-up. They cope through avoidance, attending neither the pediatric nor the adult diabetic clinic.

Some adolescents use denial or avoidance (Reid, Dulow, Carey, and Dura, 1994) in order to deal with their problem. Thus, in reference to diabetes they forget to come on time for their evening injection in order to stay with friends. They may order drinks or food that are not in their diabetic regimen in order not to be different, but to be accepted by the others and thereby escape from the feeling of shame about the self (Liakopoulou, 1994). As is evident, these self-destructive activities also serve the purpose of increasing the physical and psychological distance from the parents.

Denial is used as a defense when the adolescent ego is faced with limitations to its narcissistic aspirations (Erlich, 1986). Although it serves the process of adolescent adaptation for a limited period, in diabetes it is also associated with poor metabolic control (Reid et al., 1994). This leads the adolescent into conflict with his or her parents, and postpones the capacity to be alone and the separation process. It also postpones adaptation to the reality of diabetes, which is ever-present and needs care. Occasionally, both adolescent and parent suffer from the same illness. Blame is then attributed to the parent, usually through angry arguments and efforts to disregard parental advice. These do not help to achieve the desired psychological distance or further the individuation process. Blame, however, can be projected on parents regardless of whether or not they share the same illness, and for the adolescent it has the same consequences as mentioned above.

PROGRESSION AND REGRESSION

Although chronic illness in itself leads the adolescent to regressive steps, his innate endowment leads him to progression, to separation steps, and individuation experiences. An adolescent with adrenal hyperplasia recounted that when she was a little younger she read a lot to show off and feel superior. Although feeling superior did not help with her peer relations, her internal sense of competence held her narcissistic equilibrium in sufficiently good balance to allow her to make a forward movement, in spite of her insecurity. A late adolescent diabetic female was an excellent student at the Institute of Technology. This allowed her to have good relations with her professors, which was a positive approach to new identifications. At the same time she dared not eat a sandwich in the presence of others. With great difficulty she attended a school field trip, although she feared that the secret of her diabetes would be revealed. Maturation processes were operating in synchrony with regressive trends.

Adolescents with diabetes are encouraged to exercise regularly, and most of them do. Involvement in sports is another avenue for promoting the separation–individuation process, and improving self-esteem. At the same time these adolescents, because of their denial or their inability to control impulses, disregard the dietary demands and have poor metabolic control.

PARENTAL ANXIETIES

The personality of the parents can affect the separation process. A father with obsessive–compulsive and anxiety traits felt intense disappointment and anxiety every time his daughter's daily blood sugar was elevated. This may have affected her separation–individuation process because she stayed at home and did not want to go out with friends.

Many parents of chronically ill adolescents have a tendency to overprotect their children. The father of a diabetic midadolescent male passed by the gym to check if his son was really there and to bring him a raincoat in case it should rain. Such behavior by the father led to fights between them. Parents who promote the independence of their children prematurely with too much responsibility, may create a feeling of sadness, a sense of neglect, and loneliness in the early adolescent diabetic child. Then the youngster may feel neglected and unable to use the parents as a stable base for "emotional refueling." Anxiety in the adolescent may come to the forefront then along with sadness, and loss of metabolic control may occur.

SOCIAL CLASS

Social class may also play an important role in accelerating or delaying the separation–individuation process. Diabetic working class adolescents take on the responsibility for their insulin injections earlier than other adolescents. A 12-year-old gives himself insulin injections while his parents are at work, early in the morning or late at night. He does not perceive his parents as being neglectful or pushing him toward separation because he knows the exigencies of their reality.

New technology plays its role as well. Since an insulin syringe in the form of a fountain pen was invented, many youngsters can attend parties or go out for an uninterrupted evening with friends. With this arrangement peer contacts may continue without unpleasant inquiries or comments, which could lead to feelings of shame. The possibility of new identifications and psychological distancing from parents thus becomes real.

Acceptance of diabetes takes place during the late teens (Holmes, 1983). Before this, the adolescent has to mourn the loss of a healthy body state. "Only through a process of mourning can one become free of his constant struggle with the disability," writes Szalita (1964), and adds:

Through the process of mourning one may achieve a state of calm, become capable of making a distinction between one's self and the disability. The disability then becomes depersonalized. We no longer have two persons: there is one with a more or less limited equipment. I would not call such a state acceptance of the disability . . . there is nothing acceptable about a disability; at best one may become dispassionate about it [p. 481].

The psychiatrist who follows chronically ill adolescents has to assist them through this process of mourning. If this is successful in the case of diabetes, there is a twofold effect. It improves the mental state of the adolescent and also quite frequently the metabolic control. Near the end of this mourning process two of my patients with diabetes and a depressive reaction, a young man and a young woman, made the following statements. One said: "I learned to accept things as they are." "I understood that this is the only body I have, and I have to take care of it," said the other.

Treatment Strategies

Intervention on multiple levels of family functioning seems at times to be necessary in order for the adolescent to be able to start the separation and individuation process.

Case Illustration 1

Ann, a 14-year-old girl, who was pleasant, pretty, and a very good student, had difficulties in regulating her diabetes, leading to frequent fluctuations in blood glucose values. She was the only child of a foreign-born mother and a sailor father who was absent for many years of Ann's life. Now the father had a regular job near his family. Ann had a close relationship with her mother and was her mother's closest companion and confidante. She tried to satisfy both parents' desires to be an excellent student, and a tidy and obedient girl.

At that time, our intervention had two targets: mother and daughter. On examination, the mother had a number of depressive features which constituted a depressive episode. She also felt lonely in a foreign country in which she had not been able to adapt well and was angry at her husband. In treatment, the mother had the opportunity to talk about her loneliness, difficulty in communicating with her husband, and anxiety regarding

Ann's unstable diabetes. Antidepressant medication was added to her treatment, and an effort was made to mobilize her toward socialization. This succeeded to some extent. We also saw Ann's father, who came reluctantly, but agreed to make an effort to support his wife.

Ann was treated individually. Her anxiety about school was obviously connected with her wish to satisfy her parents' desire to be a good student, and her anxiety about diabetes was obviously increased out of identification with her mother. She was encouraged to exercise more, and gradually metabolic control was achieved.

Two years later, Ann's diabetes was out of control again. At that point she was very angry with both her parents. She went out much more often than before, adopted a style of dress very much different from her parents' wishes—black outfits and ragged jeans—and did not maintain her previous academic standards. She was also injecting insulin to lower her blood sugar and therefore to be able to eat more whenever she went out with friends. This initiative, to some extent in the service of individuation, led to an emergency hospitalization due to insulin coma. Then Ann described her boredom at school and at home, her irritation with her best girl friend who was giving her attention to a boyfriend, her rage at both parents, but particularly at her father with whom she had difficulties in communicating. It seemed that the need for separation from her internal objects through debasing and rejecting them had led her to a stage of alienation (Blos, 1967).

In family sessions they were able to express their anger, anxieties, and disappointment with each other. In particular, Ann discussed her need to express her independence through dressing differently and staying out for longer periods of time. Somewhat looser family rules were laid down and through Ann's insistence the parents started some activities together. During her treatment Ann expressed her loneliness, but also her determination to be more independent and not so close to her mother, her need for a boyfriend, but also her fear of being rejected. Her parents were helped in separate sessions to be more understanding and patient with her, and to look into their own marital relationship whose dysfunction distressed Ann. Gradually, the family tension abated, although there were occasional flare-ups.

Ann's separateness became better established in relation to her family, and particularly to her mother. This independence was at first achieved at the expense of metabolic control. After intervention, her diabetes was again better regulated with occasional relapses at times when she decided to go on a diet in order to lose weight. She could now accept, emotionally and intellectually, that her best girl friend would not forget her when she was devoting time to her boyfriend. Thus, regression seemed to be followed by progression in this case where family, couple, and individual interventions were utilized and appeared to be of great value. It should be emphasized that Ann's need for separation finally led her to a forward movement in spite of the difficulties posed by diabetes and her mother's dependency needs.

Counseling the parents to control their separation anxiety and allow their adolescent children to try new things, in spite of the fear of hypoglycemia, is a treatment strategy which has been helpful to the adolescent's development. The mother of a 14-year-old female was helped to allow her daughter to take the bus with some friends to a nearby town. She also allowed her to go on a short sea trip with her school without escorting her. It is not easy for parents to relinquish control since they fear that in case of an accident, they will have to deal with their own remorse and the criticism of others.

In working with adolescents with chronic physical illness, a major task and goal of the psychiatrist is to assist them in their separation–individuation process. After talking with a 13-year-old diabetic girl, who had a serious anxiety reaction before an athletic competition, we decided that her parents should not be near her during the event. As long as she was near them she was a crybaby; when the parents kept away, she was able to exercise her ego capacity for control in a much better way. This delineation of limits between self and parents helped in the separation–individuation process (Berati, 1991).

COUNTERTRANSFERENCE ISSUES

The therapist who tries to help adolescents with chronic illness and problems of individuation is frequently viewed by them as a parent who is either overly supportive, or helpless and angry. The following examples illustrate this observation.

CASE ILLUSTRATION 2

Elaine, a pretty 15-year-old girl of normal weight, had been followed at the diabetic clinic since the onset of diabetes at age 3 years. She was the youngest child in a family with older parents and two siblings in their midtwenties. When first seen at age 5, she was an attractive and bright girl, but very oppositional. Her parents complained about their difficulty setting limits due to fear that her diabetes would get worse. Review of the past history revealed that her separation–individuation process had been adversely affected due to several factors: her temperament (a moderately difficult child); as the youngest in the family the adults easily satisfied her needs, and allowed an unimpeded sense of omnipotence to emerge in her; and diabetes. Oedipal issues seemed to be at the forefront at the time of the first session.

Our intervention focused on helping her father to be able to set limits, and her mother to be less antagonistic. During late latency and preadolescence her oppositional quality subsided to a manageable degree. An older sister became a good mother substitute for her, which helped Elaine significantly.

At age 15, Elaine was again oppositional, noncompliant with her diabetic regimen, and dieting since she considered herself heavy. Her father, who was afraid of an insulin reaction, appeared to be despondent and sleepless. Her mother felt angry and helpless. Her older sister no longer had any influence on her.

In the session Elaine was impertinent, and insisted she would do whatever she liked. She appeared to be affirming her separateness regressively. The psychiatrist's sense of omnipotence was challenged and she felt like a helpless mother with angry feelings.

In the following session her psychiatrist, who was aware of the countertransference feelings, tried to empathize with Elaine, to understand her anxiety about the possibility of not being as likeable, or as ideally pretty as she wanted, and being fearful of rejection by boys. To put it differently, the focus was on Elaine's need for differentiation from her mother, who was moderately overweight, and her need for individuation.

In subsequent sessions she was helped to see that she could find ways to satisfy her impulses, but also to take care of her diabetes which did not need to be an obstacle to her desires. In this way, her ego was supported and reality testing could be used more effectively. Control of the therapist's countertransference feelings and the use of empathy helped Elaine's treatment and supported her development. Her mother was seen in parallel and encouraged to change her attitude from being highly critical, to being more supportive and compromising.

CASE ILLUSTRATION 3

Issues concerning identity formation, ego boundaries, separation, individuation, and countertransference, as they were intertwined with the effects of chronic illness, are illustrated in the following case.

Eva, a 19-year-old woman with congenital adrenal hyperplasia, was referred from the Endocrine Clinic because of her moodiness and inability to mobilize herself. She was on daily replacement treatment with corticosteroids. She was pretty and very intelligent, and a sophomore in French liberal studies at the university. Her investment in the courses was minimal and she doubted the correctness of her choice. She had some friends at school but she felt some of them were snobbish to her.

Her middle-class family, which consisted of mother, father, and an older brother, was very warm and understanding toward her. They tended to indulge her demands and accept her complaints because of her illness. The relationship with her brother was very close and she talked with him for hours at home. Thus, she

avoided the need to be with another man, and to make a heterosexual object choice. Eva's clinical picture was that of dysthymia
without suicidal ideation.

Despite her behavior of feigning independence she seemed to
have difficulty separating from her family, as was evident from
her fluctuating attachment to friends, and tendency to isolate
when others were critical of her. In her sessions she complained,
described her changing moods, and found understanding. Her
perceptiveness and imaginative way of describing her experiences
made her a "special daughter" for the therapist in the same way
she was for her family.

In the course of her summer vacation with her friends, her
difficulties surfaced even more. She allowed herself to regress at
times. She "forgot" to take her daily medication, thus risking
dehydration and electrolyte imbalance. One night, without medication and after some drinks and dancing at a tavern, she separated from her friends, but in the presence of a young man whom
"she detested," she fainted. In the morning she found herself in
bed with the young man who made sexual advances. In discussing
the episode Eva expressed sadness about what had happened,
and anger at the young man. "Forgetting" her medication was
examined, and the possibility that she was trying to forget that
she was different from the others was interpreted. She said that
nothing had happened previously when she forgot her medication and that she was used to having her mother remind her to
take it. She avoided acknowledging that she could have protected
herself by taking the necessary precautions. Of course, we kept
in mind the probability that she did not want to protect herself,
hoping to see, in her inebriated state, whether she was accepted
by a man. After empathizing with her, I felt it was necessary to
differentiate myself from her position of denial, and challenge
the defense of this "special child." I told her that it would have
been possible to take responsibility for herself and not to allocate
it to others like the young man on vacation, or her mother at
home; but something prevented her from doing it. She was dissatisfied with me and resisted my interpretation, but she admitted
that she had a hard time accepting herself. Some time later she

went as an exchange student to Spain for a semester, in an attempt to separate from her family and to individuate. She wrote back saying that this new experience was helping her mature.

CONCLUSION

Separation and individuation is not a smooth process for many adolescents. Chronic physical illness slows down the separation–individuation process of adolescents, but not in a uniform way. Our observations, as well as those of others, indicated to us that the innate push toward separation and individuation becomes apparent in a number of ways, and despite the regressions which take place, a forward movement occurs. The nature of the illness, the innate endowment of the youngster, the quality of the defenses, social class, technology, and most importantly parents, play their role in promoting or delaying this process. Mental health professionals can assist adolescents and their parents to avoid lengthy and regressive periods while this process is at work. Countertransference issues can be an obstacle in working with these adolescents and have to be addressed.

REFERENCES

Berati, S. (1991), Object relations in adolescence. *Psychiatriki,* 2:131–135.
Blos, P. (1967), The second individuation process of adolescence. *The Psychoanalytic Study of the Child,* 22:162–186. New York: International Universities Press.
Capelli, M., McGrath, P., Heck, C., McDonald, N., Feldman, W., & Rowe P. (1989), Chronic disease and impact. The adolescent's perspective. *J. Adol. Health Care,* 10:283–288.
Eiser, C. (1990), Psychological effects of chronic disease, *J. Child Psychol. Psychiat.,* 31:85–98.
Erikson, E. (1950), *Childhood and Society.* New York: W. W. Norton.
Erlich, H. S. (1986), Denial in adolescence. *The Psychoanalytic Study of the Child,* 41:315–336. New Haven, CT: Yale University Press.

Holmes, D. (1983), Diabetes in its psychosocial context. In: *Joslin's Diabetes Mellitus,* ed. A. Marble, L. P. Krall, R. F. Bradley, A. R. Christlieb, & J. S. Solldner. Philadelphia: Lea & Febiger, pp. 882–905.

Isay, R. (1977), The second separation stage of adolescence. In: *The Course of Life: Adolescence,* Vol. 4, ed. S. Greenspan & G. Pollock. Madison, CT: International Universities Press, pp. 457–467.

Jacobson, A. M., Hauser, S. T., Lavori, P., Wolfsdorf, J. I., Herskowitz, R. D., Millet, J. E., Bliss, R., & Gelfand, E. (1990), Adherence among children and adolescents with insulin-dependent diabetes mellitus over a four year longitudinal follow-up: 1. The influence of patient coping and adjustment. *J. Ped. Psychol.,* 15:511–526.

Kashani, J. H., Koenig, P., Shepperd, J. A., Whilfley, D., & Morris, D. A. (1988), Psychopathology and self-concept in asthmatic children. *J. Ped. Psychol.,* 13:509–520.

Liakopoulou, M., (1994), The self-esteem of the adolescent with diabetes. In: *Adolescence: The Mirror of Transition,* ed. J. Tsiantis, K. Christianopoulos, D. Anastasopoulos, M. Liakopoulou, & B. Chanzara. Athens: Kastaniotis Publications, pp. 201–207.

Mahler, M. (1968), *On Human Symbiosis and the Vicissitudes of Individuation.* New York: International Universities Press, pp. 7–31.

—— (1972), On the first three subphases of the separation–individuation process. *Internat. J. Psycho-Anal.,* 53:333–338.

—— Pine, F., & Bergman, A. (1975), *The Psychological Birth of the Human Infant.* New York: Basic Books.

Miller, A. (1973), Identification and adolescent development. In: *Adolescent Psychiatry,* Vol. 2. New York: Basic Books, pp. 199–210.

Moran, G. S. (1984), Psychoanalytic treatment of diabetic adolescents. *The Psychoanalytic Study of the Child,* 39:407–447. New Haven, CT: Yale University Press.

Reid, G., Dulow, E., Carey, T., & Dura, J. (1994), Contribution of coping to medical adjustment and treatment responsibility among children and adolescents with diabetes. *Develop. Behav. Ped.,* 15:327–335.

Rovet, J. F., Erlich, R. M., & Hope, M. (1987), Intellectual deficits associated with early onset insulin-dependent diabetes mellitus in children. *Diabetes Care,* 10:510–515.

Rutter, M., Tizard, J., & Whitmore, K. (1970), *Education, Health and Behavior.* London: Longmans.

Spirito, A., Stark, L., Gil, K., & Tyc, V. (1995), Coping with every-day and disease related stressors by chronically ill children and adolescents. *J. Amer. Acad. Child Adolesc. Psychiatry,* 33:283–290.

Szalita, A. B. (1964), De fysisk handicappede. *Nordisk Psychiatrisk Tidskrift,* 18:479–484.

Ungerer, J., Horgan, B., Chaitow, J., & Champion, G. B. (1988), Psychosocial functioning in children and young adults with juvenile arthritis. *Pediatrics,* 8:195–202.

6

Difficulties Encountered by Adolescent Thalassemia Patients

DIONYSIA PANITZ, DIPL.PSYCH.

There is an extensive literature on the psychosocial impact of chronic illness in which most authors refer to the implications of chronic illness on the development of children, and in particular its effects on the emotional, social, and cognitive levels (Pless and Rophmann, 1971; Raimbault, 1973; Zeltrer, Kellerman, Ellenberg, Dash, and Rigler, 1980; Eiser, 1985). More recently, emphasis has been given to the adjustment of the child and the family to the physical disorder, which has also been related to specific coping and defense strategies. Determinants of coping include disease-related factors (severity, chronicity); intrapersonal factors (age, personality, intelligence); and environmental factors (family communication and interaction) (Lipowski, 1970; Pless and Pinkerton, 1975; Lavigne and Burns, 1981).

Some authors even propose that illness and disability may have positive effects on some aspects of adjustment and personality development (Stein and Jessop, 1984; Georganda, 1990). Thus, children with chronic illness and their families may display various reactions following diagnosis and cannot be considered as a homogeneous group (Eiser, 1985).

109

Thalassemia

Beta-thalassemia, also known as Cooley's anemia or Mediterranean anemia, is a congenital, potentially lethal illness, inherited through asymptomatic carriers in a Mendelian, recessive manner. It is endemic in southern Europe and the tropics, but as a result of migration it has now spread throughout Europe. It ranks among the most common inherited diseases in many urban areas, and in southern Europe up to 19 percent of the population in some areas have the thalassemia trait (World Health Organization, 1988).

The thalassemia trait is commonly called *stigma* in Greece. This implies that the whole family can be stigmatized by the presence of the illness (Georganda, 1988). The diagnosis is usually made during the first months of life. Children with beta-thalassemia suffer from a chronic form of hemolytic anemia which calls for frequent blood transfusions, usually twice a month, as well as the regular administration of iron chelating agents to prevent hemosiderosis. Chelation therapy is a daily treatment administrated at home, by subcutaneous infusion using a portable pump over 8 to 10 hours, usually during the night. Such treatment has increased the average life expectancy of these children, from the first up until and including the third decade of life. Moreover, properly treated patients, as a rule, do not appear markedly different from their healthy peers.

In untreated or inproperly treated patients, physical function is considerably impaired, and clinical features are impressive. They have considerable stunting of growth, gross bone deformities, severe anemia, malnutrition, weakness, and enlargement of the spleen and liver (Kattamis, 1977). Many young adults, due to inadequate treatment in childhood, manifest several of the above features. Furthermore, the lifelong transfusions may be complicated by the effects of hemosiderosis, such as diabetes, liver and heart disease, as well as by serious infections (hepatitis-B, AIDS, and more recently hepatitis-C). These are major hazards for these patients, and impose severe restrictions on their daily life.

Our clinical observations are derived from the psychosocial support programs for thalassemic patients, who are followed up by the Thalassemia Unit of the First University Pediatric Clinic and the corresponding Unit of the National Health System at the Aghia Sophia Children's Hospital. The total number of patients monitored is approximately 1100. These patients come both from Athens and the provinces. They range from infants to 30-year-olds.

PSYCHOLOGICAL EFFECTS OF THALASSEMIA

There are only a few studies on psychiatric disturbances in thalassemic children and adolescents, although the literature does refer to the psychological problems encountered by these children and adolescents, as well as the emotional reactions and difficulties of their parents (Matsaniotis, 1973; Papadakou-Lagogianni, Xypolyta-Tsantili and Tsiantis, 1979; Tsiantis, Xypolyta-Tsantili, and Papadakou-Lagogianni, 1982; Massaglia, Pozzan, Pipa, Davico, Luzzato, and Carpignano, 1986; Piperia, Sotiropoulou, Assimopoulos, and Anastasopoulos, 1988; Pitsouni, Boura, des Lingeris, Karagiorga, Ladis, and Tsiantis, 1990).

Among the more systematic research projects carried out in this field is that of Logothetis, Haritos-Fatouros, Constantanlakis, Economidou, Augustakis, and Loewenson (1971), who reported that a significant number of patients displayed behavior and personality disturbances such as impulsiveness, temper tantrums, withdrawal, and increased dependency. Depression occurred in 50 percent of the cases.

When Tsiantis (1984) studied the mental disturbances and intelligence among children with beta-thalassemia, he found that these children displayed a high incidence of psychiatric symptoms, with neurosis and anxiety the most frequent diagnoses, followed by depression. Furthermore, he stressed that the patients

often display psychosomatic symptoms. In the preschool and latency stages they usually are anxious and tend to be overdepen-
dent on their parents. The assessment of personality revealed that
the defense mechanisms of denial and displacement were used
more often by these children, which was confirmed by Pitsouni
et al. (1990) in thalassemic adolescents. Tsiantis (1984) noted
that the intellectual functioning of children with beta-thalassemia
seems not to be affected by the illness.

There are even fewer studies on the psychological effects of
thalassemia on adolescents and young adults. Perhaps the reason
for this is that until recently thalassemia was viewed as a disease
of childhood since death usually occurred before adulthood. It
has been suggested that thalassemic adolescents encounter difficulties in relationships with their peers and are often socially
isolated, especially when they differ from their peers in their physical appearance (Tsiantis, 1990). In a recent study Zani, Di Palma,
and Vullo (1995) found that the illness does not necessarily exert
an adverse effect on the psychosocial development of thalassemic
adolescents. On the contrary, they suggest that the improved
medical care associated with adequate psychosocial support offered at their center resulted in improved social adjustment and
self-esteem for thalassemic adolescents. According to the authors
this implies that thalassemic adolescents who are helped to develop coping strategies and appropriate defense mechanisms,
may manage to adjust socially and acquire a satisfactory quality
of life.

PARENTAL ASPECTS

The parents of thalassemic children are usually described as overprotective, guilty, and self-blaming. Self-blame is associated with
the hereditary nature of the illness, and its transmission from
them to the child (Georganda, 1988). Many parents find it very
difficult to come to terms with the disease, and deny it. They
hardly talk about the illness in the family and avoid providing
information or explanations to the patient. Often parents lie
about the nature of the disease and the treatment requirements,

thus creating misconceptions and a conspiracy of silence around the problem (Tsiantis, Anastasopoulos, Meyer, Panitz, Ladis, Platokouki, Aroni, and Kattamis, 1990). Also, parents make great efforts to hide the diagnosis from relatives and friends, giving rise to a sense of shame in the patient (Tsiantis et al., 1982; Massaglia et al., 1986; Georganda, 1988; Piperia et al., 1988).

<h3>TREATMENT ASPECTS</h3>

There are some specific and crucial issues in thalassemia which characterize its emotional impact as a chronic disease. First of all, the daily chelation therapy, which is very painful, has to be done at home by the parents beginning when the child is young. Later on, the adolescent is asked to take over this responsibility. The "making of a hole" with the needle to insert the pump (Massaglia and Carpignano, 1987), implies a daily aggressive act directed against the ill body, and is a reminder of the illness. Fears of complications and the threat of premature death, hinder the use of repression, keeping death fear on a conscious level.

Growing up is feared by adolescent patients since the illusion of cure diminishes with age, and there is the threat of a sudden complication which can lead to death. This constant threat preoccupies adolescents and interferes with the need to deal with the demands of normal development. Thalassemic patients are not only dependent on the help of their parents for their treatment needs, but also on their doctors, the hospital, and blood donors. Such massive dependency in adolescence involves ambivalence and arouses aggression.

<h3>REACTIONS TO THE INITIAL DIAGNOSIS</h3>

The diagnosis of thalassemia in their child is usually experienced by the parents as a narcissistic trauma which concerns their potency and adequacy. They usually try to hide the illness from the social environment to avoid stigmatization with its repetitive narcissistic mortification. This aspect is illuminated in Greek mythology when Hera dropped Hephaestus from the top of Mount

Olympus because of the narcissistic mortification which his birth caused her. According to the myth, Hephaestus, the smith-god, was born ugly, weak, and ill-tempered. In another version of the myth he was handicapped with a limp in one leg. This disgusted his mother, Hera, who tried to rid herself of the embarrassment it caused her. When Hera was informed later about his workmanship, she called him back to Olympus and arranged for him to marry Aphrodite, the goddess of beauty. Since Aphrodite symbolizes perfection of the body, the gift of Hera can be understood as a reparative gesture offering Hephaestus a complement for his handicapped body.

Returning to the point of the initial diagnosis of thalassemia, the following issues could be raised: How does the illness affect the parental view of the child? Are its implications overwhelming to the ego of the mother-child or is the distress manageable? How does it influence the separation–individuation process? What are the vicissitudes of body image development up to this point, and how does it influence the subsequent development of the body image?

ASPECTS OF THE MOTHER–CHILD RELATIONSHIP

We might suppose that the impact of the illness on the early mother–child relationship, depending on the age at which the condition is noted, has certain serious implications on the structuring of narcissism. This is decisive for the nature of the relationship between ego, ego ideal, and the external objects. Regarding self-object differentiation, we might further suppose that a diagnosis of chronic illness also has certain implications for the separation–individuation process and the resulting autonomy of the child. Under the stress of illness the child is more vulnerable to regression along the continuum of self-object differentiation. Children with thalassemia seem not to succeed in separating from their mothers, and usually remain dependent in a close, ambivalent relationship to both parents.

Effects on Body Image

Regarding body image development, Freud (1923, p. 26) wrote that the ego is first and foremost a bodily ego. The body ego is built up through the care of the infant by his mother. Winnicott (1971) described the child looking at his mother's face and seeing a reflection of himself, in other words, mirroring himself in the eyes of his mother. This mirror image is then incorporated into the body image and ultimately into the self-concept. In this way, the esteem of one's body will become an essential part of self-esteem. A diagnosis of chronic illness breaks the mirror, at least for a time. The child looks at the face of the mother to mirror him- or herself and becomes confused. The child studies the mirror to find some sense of themselves. According to Winnicott (1971), if there is a defect or illness in the child and a corresponding narcissistic defect or illness in the mother, she is often unable to accept this and reflect back to the child his or her true and intact body image. Thus, the child's body image remains undeveloped, or becomes distorted by narcissistic defenses.

The Adolescent Process in Thalassemia

On reaching adolescence, according to Blos (1962), a second individuation process takes place. A second chance is offered, or a second trauma occurs if the process miscarries. For thalassemic adolescents, restrictions imposed by the illness and dependency (on blood donors, on the usually overprotective parent, and on physicians) are obstacles in the way of the normal process of acquiring autonomy. As a result, the second individuation process cannot be achieved. Thus, the thalassemic adolescent remains dependent and highly ambivalent toward the parents.

On addressing the issues of the final development of body image and sexuality, we have to take into consideration that ego development is particularly evident with emancipation of the body from parental (especially maternal) control, care, and protection. Then there accrues a sense of total ownership of the body, which the thalassemic youngster fails to experience. More-over, physical sexual maturity, which normally takes place in ado-lescence, means a fundamental change in the person's relationship to his or her body. It may happen that the sexual body arouses fear, which can result in regression to the idealized prepubertal body image.

In the thalassemic adolescent the secondary sexual characteris-tics, including endocrine, do not occur, or are delayed and in-complete because of the deficiency of the endocrine glands. The immature body, lacking secondary sexual characteristics, to-gether with delayed and unsatisfactory skeletal growth, and an inadequate individuation process, affects the final establishment of body image and sexuality. If the illness has until now been a family secret, the adolescent will now be confronted with the fact that his/her appearance differs from that of peers, and he/she is suspected of being ill. We have to bear in mind that the thalasse-mic adolescent has experienced repeated, traumatic, and over-whelming assaults on his or her body boundaries resulting in a body image that has been poorly integrated. As the body repeat-edly becomes a source of disappointment, anxiety, and psychic pain, castration feelings emerge with difficulties in integrating the body image into the personality organization. Thalassemic adolescents may defend themselves and try to improve their self-esteem either by splitting off the often distorted body image, or by denying the conflict. Such an effort may lead to breaches with reality.

In consideration of the above issues, against the backdrop of their chronic illness, adolescence may constitute another trauma for thalassemic patients.

CASE ILLUSTRATION

Several of these issues will be demonstrated in the case of Dimitris, a thalassemic 17-year-old. He refused transfusion and ran away from the hospital unit. He was often uncooperative with the clinical staff, noncompliant with treatment, and expressed suicidal thoughts by saying that he was "going to leave."

He was an intelligent, short adolescent who lacked secondary sex characteristics and thus appeared much younger than his peers. He was rather quiet, with an angry expression and depressed mood. His attitude toward his parents and doctors was characterized by constant opposition.

His father was a retired salesman, and his mother was a housewife, devoted to his care and treatment needs. After the diagnosis was made the parents decided not to tell anybody about the illness. Thus, Dimitris was forced to lie in school, to friends, and neighbors. The parents had many misconceptions about the nature of the illness and its possible physical and emotional effects.

Dimitris felt misunderstood by his parents, and especially his father, who did not take him seriously, and laughed at his shame about his childish appearance. He was left alone to carry the heavy burden of his illness. Further, he felt that he was a source of shame for the family and that they wanted to get rid of him. Thus, he never felt accepted and loved, and could not accept his diagnosis or adjust to the idea of having to live with a chronic disease. He always felt different from other people, and that he was "a cripple." The major source of disappointment was his body which he hated, since in his view, it was the obstacle to his life as a sexual young adult. He expressed his negative attitude about his body by describing how, in chelation therapy, he "pins the pump into his belly with hate."

He perceived people treating him as a child, although he was a young adult, and complained that girls lacked interest in a heterosexual relationship with him. He was depressed, and believed that nobody, and nothing, could help him to reverse his illness. He decided never to accept life as a cripple. Although he stated that psychotherapy could not change anything either, he never missed his sessions, and used them to express his thoughts and feelings. After a year of weekly therapy (while a colleague saw his parents), he decided to postpone his decision to commit suicide. He used my care and interest, and that of the medical staff, as a motive to continue life, "for our sake," he said. Despite that, he had not given up his plan to get rid of his body. "I'm already familiar with this idea," he said, "it does not scare me anymore. I believe in the immortality of the soul. I will get rid of my disgusting body. It is only a question of time. In this way I will stop suffering." At the same time he accepted treatment with hormones (substitution therapy), but became disappointed with the failure to develop secondary sexual characteristics. He also complained about the restrictions imposed on him because of the additional complication of diabetes.

On working through his feelings about his illness, the treatment, and the hospital admissions, he mentioned that he always carried a knife with him as a defense when he came to the hospital. At the same time he was afraid of losing control and using it. This could possibly happen if somebody from the clinical staff asked him to accept a treatment he did not wish, or hindered him when he wanted to leave the hospital. He could link being armed with a weapon to his feeling of being "unarmed" against the intrusion by the transfusions and other treatment requirements. We understood that his hostility, mainly directed against his parents, who had transmitted the disease and were, in his opinion, unavailable to share the burden with him, was displaced and turned against himself, especially against his body, which was the source of all somatic and psychic pain.

He referred to Sparta and the attitude of Spartans toward sick and weak children. In ancient Greece, Sparta was the city with the best soldiers. To have the right to become a citizen of Sparta a man had to be healthy and able-bodied. Spartan mothers threw their weak, sick, or handicapped children off a cliff into Keadas. He stated that this was what his parents should have done when he was diagnosed, but he would do it himself. Suicide was, in his opinion, an act of Spartan bravery.

Similar material appeared in his suicidal fantasies. He thought of throwing himself off a terrace to be smashed. With this act he would, in his fantasy, undo his condition and the "cripple" would become a brave Spartan. At the same time he was identifying with the aggressor, the Spartan mother, sacrificing part of himself, his body, to save the whole, the self.

Working through the context of his thoughts and fantasies, and as the transference relationship became established, he decided to continue his life as a youngster with thalassemia, under the condition that he would never accept additional treatment or hospitalization. A possible complication of his illness would be the millstone which he would never accept. He stated that he hated the hospital as much as he hated his body, and considered it to be a dirty place which only caused him pain and depression.

A specific area of interest which helped Dimitris through the depressive periods was history. He was supported in therapy to expand his interests since this seemed to enrich his psychic life. He enjoyed reading historical documents and became impressed with the Third Reich. He admired the *Schutzstaffel* (SS). He shared the ideology of the Aryan race, and described in detail the healthy, robust, and strong bodies of the soldiers. He did not believe they had committed the crimes of which they were accused. In his eyes this battalion was pure and proper. In confrontation with reality, he used denial. We may suppose that the real events threw a shadow over his ideal and in order to preserve it, he denied reality. At the same time he was able to recognize that he possibly would have become their victim. Identifying once again with the aggressor, he found it reasonable to become a target for extermination. All these themes contained self-destructiveness and were worked through in therapy. His effort to sacrifice his body to rescue his soul was a central theme repeated in his thoughts and fantasies.

Later on, Dimitris found a better balance and began to enjoy his life. He entered the university to study history, which was a source of pleasure for him. He met new peers and became interested in music and traveling. Although he seemed to feel much better, his attitude toward treatment remained basically unchanged.

The work with the parents did not follow a parallel path with Dimitris' therapy. The parents, who where of a lower educational

level and less psychologically minded than their son, had difficulty in finding a way to communicate with him. Despite the
therapist's efforts, they found it hard to understand, accept, and
share the burden of his illness. They tried to distance themselves
from Dimitris' difficulties and avoided cooperating in counseling.

The fragile psychic balance that Dimitris had achieved lasted
for two years. Then, one day he came to the Unit with a high
fever, and his doctors thought he had simply caught a cold. His
condition worsened rapidly, but he denied that he had to be
treated. The staff and his parents tried to persuade him to cooper-
ate and enter the adult hospital. I was asked to support him in
this decision, and he was finally sent there by ambulance. A few
days later we learned that Dimitris was dead. He had not accepted
hospitalization, insisting on going home, and had died of acute
meningitis, before the diagnosis could be made.

DISCUSSION

Dimitris' difficulties were related to the demands placed on him
by his chronic illness, and especially during adolescence by the
changing body, which failed to develop sexually. His distorted
body image caused a breach with reality. His ego became overwhelmed by the difficulties imposed on it by the illness, which
were barely manageable and were experienced as traumatic. The
ego ideal content of the SS and the idealized bodies of the soldiers
can be understood as an effort to establish an ideal, or a "pseudo-
ideal," according to Laufer (1964). This ego ideal, as part of a
harsh superego, was directed against the ego, which tried to integrate by splitting into the body ego and the psychic ego. Thus,
aggression was turned against the body so that the psyche could
survive. His sudden terminal illness, requiring numerous clinical
examinations and hospitalization, threatened him with regression
and anxieties from the past. His integration seemed to weaken,
which led to his decision to refuse treatment and hospitalization.

This can be understood as a suicidal act, which in fantasy was turned only against his body ego, but in reality caused his biological death.

The aim of the psychotherapeutic work was primarily ego supportive. Dimitris was helped to gain a better understanding of his disease, with a more realistic perspective, including its restrictions and possibilities. He was further supported in his efforts to take on more responsibility for his treatment. This led to improved cooperation with the medical and nursing staff which gave him the feeling that he had some control over his illness. It resulted in greater acceptance with awareness, and not denial, of the illness, and helped him to develop some coping strategies. This gave meaning to his life in the present, while he was learning to live with the uncertainty of the future.

By expressing his thoughts and feelings and working them through, he was helped to discover new areas of interest, developing his capacities, and thereby, enriching his ego. The new experience of being listened to, and understood, made him feel less isolated. Using this experience we tried to work through the relationship with the parents, which was crucial for his present difficulties and further development. The aggression and sadomasochism which dominated this relationship, mainly in the relationship with his mother, placed him in a highly ambivalent and dependent position vis-à-vis his parents. Additionally, the requirements of his physical therapy made him feel that he was deprived of his independence. These feelings and demands counteracted the normal process of acquiring autonomy and independence in adolescence. By dealing with the patient's and parents' aggression, we hoped to find a communication path for them, which might lead Dimitris to feel accepted as a family member *with a chronic disease*. However, this goal was not accomplished in the work with the parents since they avoided the counseling offered.

In Dimitris' psychotherapy we assumed that working through these feelings might help him to resolve some of his conflicts. In regard to his available defense mechanisms, we tried to strengthen and expand his ego functions while we attempted to decrease his pathological defenses. With these efforts we hoped to enhance his bonds with life. Psychotherapy helped him to find a new, better balance and gain better understanding of his emotional conflicts, but did not succeed in reversing the course of self-destructiveness, which finally took the upper hand and led to his premature death.

CONCLUSION

The developmental periods which seem to be the most crucial in thalassemia are when the diagnosis is made, usually during the first months of the infant's life, and in adolescence. The diagnosis of thalassemia affects the whole family and has serious repercussions on the mother–child relationship, with implications for the early development of the child.

On reaching adolescence, the thalassemic patient has to deal with the normal but demanding developmental tasks of this phase, which become intensified and prolonged by the vicissitudes of the illness. These may become complicated by excess anxiety, denial, and regression.

Psychological support given to thalassemic adolescents and their parents, in the context of liaison–consultation psychiatry with the thalassemia unit, may help them resolve possible misconceptions and gain a more realistic view of their illness. This may lead to the patients' having a sense of some control over the illness. It may also promote cooperation with doctors and nursing staff, and compliance with treatment. Furthermore, psychotherapeutic intervention may strengthen the patient's ego and help to develop new defenses and coping strategies in order to come to terms with the illness. The working through of the central conflicts which most thalassemic adolescents are confronted with, such as dependency and the often distorted body image, as well as the crucial issue of premature death, may offer an opportunity for emotional growth and lead to an improved quality of life.

REFERENCES

Blos, P. (1962), *On Adolescence.* New York: Free Press.

Eiser, C. (1985), *The Psychology of Childhood Illness.* New York: Springer-Verlag.

Freud, S. (1923), The Ego and the Id. *Standard Edition,* 19:1–59. London: Hogarth Press, 1961.

Georganda, E. T. (1988), Thalassemia and the adolescent: An investigation of chronic illness, individuals and systems. *Fam. Systems Med.,* 6:150–161.

—— (1990), The impact of thalassemia on body image, self-image, and self-esteem. *Ann. NY Acad. Sci.,* 612:466–472.

Kattamis, C. (1977), Social, medical and genetic effects of the thalassaemic syndromes. *Iatriki Epitheorisi Enoplon Dynameon,* 11:112–121. (In Greek)

Laufer, M. (1964), Ego ideal and pseudo ego ideal in adolescence. *The Psychoanalytic Study of the Child,* 19:196–221. New York: International Universities Press.

Lavigne, J. V., & Burns, W. J. (1981), *Pediatric Psychology: Introduction for Pediatricians and Psychologists.* New York: Grune & Stratton.

Lipowski, Z. J. (1970), Physical illness, the individual and the coping process. *Psychiatr. Med.,* 1:91–98.

Logothetis, J., Haritos-Fatouros, M., Constantanlakis, M., Economidou, J., Augustakis, O., & Loewenson, R. (1971), Intelligence and behavioral patterns in patients with Cooley's anemia (homozygous thalassemia). *Ped.,* 48:740–744.

Massaglia, P., & Carpignano, M. (1987), Psychology of the thalassemia patient and his family. In: *Thalassaemia Today: 2nd Mediterranean Meeting on Thalassaemia,* ed. G. Sirchia & A. Zanella. Milano: Policlinico di Milano, pp. 69–79.

—— Pozzan, M. T., Pipa, A., Davico, S., Luzzato, L., & Carpignano, M. (1986), Aspetti psicologici della talasemia (Psychological aspects of thalassemia). *Ped. Med. Chr.,* 8:27–39.

Matsaniotis, N. (1973), Psychological problems of thalassemia patients and their families. *Archeio Ellinikis Ematologikis Etairias,* 2:85–87. (In Greek)

Papadakou-Lagogyanni, S., Xypolyta-Tsantili, D., & Tsiantis, I. (1979), Group counseling discussions with thalassaemic parents. Paper presented at the 17th Panhellenic Pediatric Congress, Athens, June. (In Greek)

Piperia, M., Sotiropoulou, H., Assimopoulos, H., & Anastasopoulos, D. (1988), Les adolescents atteints de b-thalassemie et leurs reactions psychologiques (Adolescents diagnosed with thalassemia and their psychological reactions). *Therapie les Cahiers de l'Enseignement Specialise,* 14:11–21.

Pitsouni, D., Boura, M., des Lingeris, J., Karagiorga, M., Ladis, V., & Tsiantis, I. (1990), Psychological responses of thalassemic adolescents on the Rorschach test. *Psychologica Themata,* 3:197–208. (In Greek)

Pless, I., & Pinkerton, P. (1975), *Chronic Childhood Disorders, Promoting Patterns of Adjustment.* London: Henry Kimpton.

—— Rophmann, K. (1971), Chronic illness and its consequences: Observations based on three epidemiological surveys. *J. Ped.,* 79:351–359.

Raimbault, G. (1973), Psychological problems in the chronic nephropathies of childhood. In: *The Child in His Family, the Impact of Disease and Death,* Vol. 2, ed. J. Anthony & C. Koupernik. New York: John Wiley.

Stein, R. E. K., & Jessop, D. J. (1984), Relationship between health status and psychological adjustment among children with chronic conditions. *Ped.,* 73:169–174.

Tsiantis, J. (1984), *Mental Disturbances and Intelligence in a Group of Children with b-Thalassemia.* Doctoral dissertation, Athens University Medical School, Athens. (In Greek)

―――― (1990), Family reactions and relationships in thalassemia. *Annals NY Acad. Sci.,* 612:451–461.

―――― Anastasopoulos, D., Meyer, M., Panitz, D., Ladis, V., Platokouki, N., Aroni, S., & Kattamis, C. (1990), A multi-level intervention approach for care of HIV-positive haemophiliac and thalassemic patients and their families. *Aids Care,* 2:253–265.

―――― Xypolita-Tsantili, D., & Papadakou-Lagogianni, S. (1982), Family reactions and their management in a parent's group with b-thalassemia. *Arch. Dis. Child.,* 57:860–863.

Winnicott, D. W. (1971), Mirror role of mother and family in child development. In: *Playing and Reality.* New York: Basic Books, pp. 112–113.

World Health Organization (1988), *The Haemoglobinopathies in Europe* (combined report of two WHO meetings). Unpublished document, Eur ICP/MCH 110, 3370v, WHO Regional Office for Europe, Copenhagen.

Zani, B., Di Palma, A., & Vullo, C. (1995), Psychosocial aspects of chronic illness in adolescents with thalassemia major. *J. Adol.,* 18:387–402.

Zeltrer, L., Kellerman, J., Ellenberg, L., Dash, J., & Rigler, D. (1980), Psychotropic effects of illness in adolescence: Impact of illness in adolescents. Crucial issues and coping styles. *J. Ped.,* 97:132–138.

7

Psychodynamic Aspects of Adolescents' Therapeutic Compliance Following a Kidney Transplant

SYLVIE PUCHEU, Ph.D., PAOLA ANTONELLI, Ph.D.,
AND SILLA M. CONSOLI, M.D.

Kidney transplantation is accepted today as the treatment of choice for persons with end-stage renal disease (ESRD) in all age groups. Compliance with the antirejection treatment with cyclosporine is vital to a transplant patient's good health. While a kidney transplant enables patients to avoid the constraints of hemodialysis and enjoy nearly full autonomy, they must scrupulously and regularly adhere to the treatment prescribed by the medical team. Therefore, in a successful transplant the therapy continues after the operation. Sometimes this is viewed as contradictory to the idea of the transplant ending the illness which patients associate with the procedure.

During adolescence, the basis of personality which began in childhood is reorganized. This reorganization is crucial to maintaining the continuity of emotional growth and establishing stable identifications. Puberty may upset the stable functioning of the personality and threaten narcissistic status. The psychodynamic processes observed during adolescence and those involved in the emotional integration of an organ transplant appear to be similar in three ways. These are: (1) Reorganization of the body image. (2) Acceptance of a new self-image. (3) Reactivation of castration anxiety and the Oedipus complex.

Adolescence and the transplantation experience imply bodily changes with consequences for self representation, among which are effects on narcissistic defenses. To become self-sufficient and an adult involves acknowledgment of parental help up to that point. Similarly, we feel that emotional integration for a transplant patient involves recognition by the recipient of the debt toward the transplant donor. This is closely connected with integration of the Oedipus complex and castration anxiety. Projective tests (the Rorschach and Thematic Apperception Tests [TAT]) may be used to provide an internal view of these processes. We aim to show that when transplant surgery occurs in adolescence, the developmental and transplant processes are amplified and may increase the problems of each.

LITERATURE REVIEW

The first studies concerning psychological and psychosocial issues after kidney transplantation in childhood and adolescence were conducted in the early 1970s, and the majority of these were primarily descriptive. Psychological aspects of nephropathy and ESRD, especially at this age, were presented (Shaben, 1993). One of the questions was, what is the meaning of waiting for an organ transplant from a cadaver?

Whenever a child or an adolescent is put on dialysis, it is a traumatic event (Becker, Igoin, and Delons, 1979; Gutton, 1985). Regression is frequently observed in such children and appears to be necessary for the child to accept medical treatment (Raimbault, 1973; Becker et al., 1979). In adolescence, aggressive demands, rebellion, and depression are more frequent, but depression is often masked by an attitude of self-assurance. Physiological factors can also contribute to mood changes (Calland,

1972). High dosages of cortisone can promote a confusional or acute psychotic state. But this medication does not directly interfere with compliance because it begins days after transplantation and must be resolved before hospital discharge.

When a psychiatric vulnerability already exists before transplantation, a specific follow-up is recommended (Leon, Baudin, and Consoli, 1990). During this period, denial seems to be the preferred defense mechanism (Becker et al., 1979; Gutton, 1985). Sometimes, this way of coping can lead to a refusal to accept the illness and its therapeutic limitations. Usually, denial is focused on associated requirements such as the dialysis regimen, other medical treatment, or compliance with the schedule.

Noncompliance is defined as a failure to follow through with medical treatment (Shaben, 1993). Several studies (Korsch, Negrete, Gardner, Weinstock, Mercer, Grushkin, and Fine, 1973; Malekzadeh, Pennisi, Vittenbogaat, Korsch, Fine, and Main, 1976; Litt and Chriskey, 1980) found that during adolescence it was more difficult to differentiate compliant from noncompliant patients. It was hypothesized that primarily because of their age and developmental stage, adolescents may be predisposed to noncompliance (Korsch et al., 1973; Korsh, Fine, and Negrete, 1978). After kidney transplant, 64 percent of adolescents were found to be more or less noncompliant with the antirejection immunosuppressive medication, although the general rate of noncompliance is 25 to 35 percent in adult kidney transplants (Ettenger, Rosenthal, Marik, Malekzadeh, Forsythe, Kamil, Salusky, and Fine, 1991).

The consequences of waiting for transplant are also important, because the patients have to cope with uncertainty and ambivalence (toward the donor). The uncertainty appears to be magnified and more distressful at specific times (Tisza, Dorsett, and Morse, 1976; Weems and Patterson, 1989; Nekolaiuchuck, 1990; Juneau, 1995). Such difficulties may arise when a patient is feeling bad, when a fellow dialysis patient receives or rejects a kidney, when a phone call concerning an available kidney is missed, or when the waiting period is lengthy and upsets expectations.

The ambivalence (Weems and Patterson, 1989) can be attributed to fear of surgery, but particularly to feelings concerning the donor. The wish for a kidney is experienced like a wish for someone to die (Juneau, 1995). After kidney transplant, patients indicate that the most stressful aspects are repeated hospitalization, fear of rejection, and the cost of immunosuppressive therapy. In adolescence the constant uncertainty of kidney rejection seemed to make young patients especially vulnerable (Juneau, 1995).

The combination of changes associated with adolescence, and a chronic condition such as transplantation, may set the stage for some of the greatest challenges that an individual will ever face (Kahn, Herndon, and Ahmadian, 1971; Shaben, 1993). The problem of steroid-induced body changes, which are particularly intense in the teens, is a frequently reported psychosocial aspect (Shaben, 1993). Some adolescent girls stop taking their immunosuppressive medication for these reasons (Kahn et al., 1971). In general, good or poor compliance has often been associated with health locus of control. Control over life dimensions, which includes control over illness, is a significant factor in psychological adjustment (Bremer, Haffly, Foxx, and Weaver, 1995). On the other hand, the belief that one's health is under one's control was associated with less depression, but only among those who had not previously experienced a failed renal transplant (Christensen, Turner, Smith, Holman, and Gregory, 1991).

Another study to identify variables that could be associated with noncompliance among renal transplant recipients, showed that recipients who reported higher stress and more depression, who coped with stress by using avoidant strategies, and who believed that health outcomes were beyond their control, were less compliant with both medication and follow-up (Frazier, Davis-Ali, and Dahl, 1994). Regression analysis revealed that stress was the strongest predictor of both medication and follow-up compliance.

School attendance, ability to work, and unemployment are also correlated with noncompliance (Chantler, Carter, Bewick, Counnagan, Cameron, Ogg, Williams, and Winder, 1980; Henning,

Tomlinson, Rigden, Haycock, and Chantler, 1988; Kiley, Lam, and Pollack, 1993). Young adults with a history of juvenile ESRD did not present a statistically significant excess of psychiatric problems compared with healthy subjects (Morton, Reynolds, Garralda, Postlethwaite, and Goh, 1994). Although the difference is small, lower self-esteem in renal patients raises the issue of whether psychiatric adjustment has been achieved at the cost of acceptance of psychosocial inferiority (Morton et al., 1994). In the same way, the development of social relationships may be disturbed. Adolescents were affected more than children with problems of low self-esteem, depression, and less social involvement (Reynolds, Garralda, Postlethwaite, and Goh, 1991; Reynolds, Morton, Garralda, Postlethwaite, and Goh, 1993). Successful transplantation seemed to have a positive influence on social development (Poznanski, Miller, Salguerro, and Kelsch, 1978; Reynolds et al., 1991).

The establishment of nonfamily peer relations facilitates the normal development of independence. Fifteen adolescents with ESRD and completed renal transplant were compared with a matched group of healthy adolescents. Self-esteem was similar in both groups, but the characteristics of the chronically ill adolescent social networks suggest that these patients may experience a high degree of social isolation (Melzer, Leadbeater, Reisman, Jaffe, and Lieberman, 1989).

Besides describing psychosocial issues after kidney transplant, psychoanalysts proposed an interpretation of the process through which patients can integrate the graft into their self representation. In this perspective, integrating a new organ implies mechanisms such as incorporation, introjection, or identification (Consoli and Bedrossian, 1979; Nekolaiuchuck, 1990; Leon et al., 1990). Three stages have been described in this integration and belong to the process of *internalization* (Castelnuovo-Tedesco, 1973). First, the transplanted organ is perceived as a foreign object. Fear of rejection is strong, and the transplant or the patient seems to be fragile. Then a partial incorporation follows, and the patient is less inclined to talk about the new organ. Finally, incorporation is complete. The kidney becomes "my" kidney and belongs from now on to the patient's body.

French psychoanalysts (Crombez and Lefebvre, 1973) suggested that the word *accorporation* would be more pertinent. According to them, in the process of graft integration, the mechanism is opposite to incorporation. First, the kidney is seen as a foreign part of the body, and then it becomes progressively a part of it. Moreover, the graft integration has also been interpreted as a progressive but discontinuous process, depending more on the previous personality (Basch, 1973; Baudin, 1989). Accepting a new organ also requires giving up a part of the body which has become nonfunctional (Consoli and Bedrossian, 1979).

Transplantation can be experienced as a recovery or a rebirth (Leon et al., 1990). In the latter case, the transplant appears to be able to restore what has been lost (i.e., employment and reproductive capacities). Illness can also be experienced as a castration, and transplantation makes sexuality possible. Because dialysis induces male impotence and female infertility, transplantation is an equivalent of "rephallicization" for a male, or "refertilization" for a female (Crombez and Lefebvre, 1973). Some authors (Gutton, 1985; Slama, 1987) have stated that with the sick adolescent, the integration of feelings about the suffering body (and the implant as well) will be a predominant factor in the adolescent process and its outcome.

From a psychoanalytic perspective, and in order to observe mental functioning and personality, projective methods (Rorschach and Thematic Apperception Test [T.A.T.]) provide interesting and pertinent views in general, and particularly in adolescence (Chabert, 1983, 1991; Brelet, 1986; Slama, 1987). The Rorschach provides a preferential means for identifying self representation, and how identity is perceived and experienced. In adolescent protocols, the quality of narcissistic defenses turned out to be essential (Chabert, 1983, 1991). The body changes involve a reorganization of self representation and identity, and narcissistic defenses are tested. A Rorschach study (Bourneuf and

Bouras, 1980) on kidney transplant adolescents showed an impoverishment of personality and an intensification of defenses against anxiety. This phenomenon is not observed with children who expressed, sometimes intensely, their anxiety and conflicts.

The T.A.T. is a good instrument with which to study oedipal problems because of its constant references to gender and/or generational differences (Brelet, 1986; Shentoub, Chabert, Azoulay, Bailly-Salin, Benfredj, Boekholt, Brelet-Foulard, Chretien, Emanuelli, Martin, Monin, Peruchon, and Serviere, 1990; Chabert, 1991) and the cards can reactivate castration anxiety. This test is also useful to evaluate the ability to cope with internal conflicts (i.e., the quality of defense mechanisms). In adolescence, the T.A.T. helps to recognize individuation and integration processes (Douville, 1987). Finally, the T.A.T. can highlight representations of object loss (Chabert, 1983).

CASE PRESENTATIONS

In the context of research to identify the psychological factors involved in compliance with therapy after a kidney transplant, two patients, aged 21, who had kidney failure earlier in adolescence, will be presented. They had hemodialysis, then transplantation, approximately two years later. One, who was successfully transplanted was compliant, while the other had a graft rejection due to noncompliance with therapy.

METHODS

Assessments were made at two different times. In the preoperative assessment, the patients completed a questionnaire on the quality of life to evaluate their perception of their physical and psychological health, hemodialysis, and social support. Their physician answered a medical questionnaire and evaluated therapeutic compliance from his point of view. Twelve months after transplantation, each patient had a semistructured interview with a psychologist to assess the patient's current state. The patient also had a self-administered questionnaire on locus of control (Levenson, 1973), the Rorschach, and the T.A.T. The physician completed another questionnaire and evaluated therapeutic compliance on each patient.

Our hypotheses were as follows: two types of attitudes should be correlated with a poor compliance: (1) when a negative dialysis experience is associated with an idealized view of transplant, that is, transplant is considered as an equivalent of recovery; (2) when there is a high degree of dependency and/or passivity toward the medical team and the patient's family during hemodialysis, the patient has secondary gain from hemodialysis and the family. These two attitudes should be associated with a narcissistic fragility, and a failure of paternal function.

The cases of Olivier and Jean-Michel may illustrate these hypotheses, and some particular of ESRD and renal transplant in adolescence when there is an identity crisis.

CASE 1

Olivier is a friendly young man whose nephropathy started at age 4 years, and he began hemodialysis at the age of 16. Two years later, Olivier was transplanted, but there was rejection due to poor compliance about nine months later. Olivier is the only child of often absent parents, and was brought up by a nanny. However, he claims a good relationship with both parents. His past is notable for parental separation, which occurred gradually and smoothly according to him. It was finally effected when he was put on dialysis. At that time he also left school because, he said, he was "overtaken by dialysis, social life, and school all at the same time."

He was very negative about being on dialysis again, even though he accepted his autodialysis rather well. He recognized that in order to face his illness and dialysis, he preferred "not to think"; "the only idea to help me to live is to be registered again on a waiting list"; "I am ready to receive a pig's kidney." He feared that dialysis would damage him.

In his transplant prequestionnaire, Olivier considered dialysis as a painful constraint to which he responded with indifference. His responses expressed total disdain for the dialysis machine, the medical treatment, his state of health, and his relationship to the medical team and other patients. He was late for dialysis. Despite the many pains accompanying these sessions, he responded to questions about his physical and moral well-being as a state of perfect health: "All is well apart from my sessions of hemodialysis. I like every other day." This general attitude of self-assurance, a kind of compensation for his precarious situation and a negation of the problems, shows the need for Olivier to present a healthy and strong image of himself at all costs.

On the Rorschach and T.A.T., Olivier was overwhelmed by castration anxiety and seemed to remain fixated on the somatic handicap.

He expressed his desire "to do away with medical dependency," and the tests confirmed his willingness to maintain an "omnipotent" position (which is in fact very precarious) to convince us and himself of his independence. Through the process of identification, the paternal image is the guardian of this heritage and its transmission. For Olivier, this image was expressed in terms of lack and absence, which is not constructive. Sometimes, it brings out poorly controlled hostility.

Since he did not have a strong and well-defined paternal image, relationships might stimulate too much anxiety for him. We could understand better, then, his difficulty in collaborating with his doctors. The person he needs is also dangerous, and his debt becomes unbearable. Referring to illegal organ traffic, Olivier said: "I cannot bear to pay someone for this." Olivier is handicapped by intense anxiety and a poor self-image.

CASE 2

Jean-Michel's nephropathy began at age 17, and hemodialysis started immediately. His illness did not seem to affect his studies, which were already quite poor since he left school at 14. He has not yet made a vocational choice, and this preoccupies him currently. He is the third of five children. Jean-Michel is rather shy, lonely, and without friends, but he is very close to his family. To him, the transplant means more free time and freedom, despite no change in his relationships.

His questionnaire before transplantation showed that he considered dialysis therapeutic and a contribution to his well-being. If there are limits, they seem well-accepted. He scrupulously observed the treatment schedule, and felt no pain during the sessions. Jean-Michel used the treatment time to draw and read. It was a reassuring time to him. Jean-Michel could integrate and turn his body preoccupation into an active constructive behavior. The confrontation with castration anxiety seemed not to be overwhelming, and he managed it with detachment. Relationships were reassuring and used as positive support.

The psychological tests, and particularly the projective tests, confirmed the dynamics and richness of his ability to cope with different conflicts, due to managing his oedipal conflict appropriately. This probably explains the acceptance of the pseudocastration via transplantation.

A year after his operation he preferred not to mention the transplant or the donor, even if "he thinks of them often." He had a sort of secret relationship with the donor. This stage of graft integration is frequent in successful transplantation. In Jean-Michel's case, this could be attributed to the quality of his defense mechanisms.

The two following examples are particularly significant: with the T.A.T. card which suggests two masculine figures, one young and one older, symbolizing the relationship of father and son, Jean-Michel concludes: "There is something that may be used in what they have learned (the older ones). We can learn a lot from them but also vice versa." Jean-Michel seemed able to identify himself with a positive paternal image. Accepting such an identification enabled him to integrate his own personality without conflict. The same was seen with the card symbolizing archaic thinking about which he commented: his "visit to the mountain. . . . Petit Jean decides to take some pictures. . . . He sees a quarry, decides to examine the stones, and brings some to his professor so that he can tell him about them. Thanks to that, he passes his exams and is rewarded."

DISCUSSION

Illness interfered with Olivier's school attendance, but not Jean-Michel's, and contributed to unemployment and relative social isolation for both youngsters (Chantler et al., 1980; Henning et al., 1988; Melzer et al., 1989; Kiley et al., 1993; Reynolds et al., 1991, 1993). In Olivier's case, poor peer relations have been exaggerated by the absence of "normal" life during childhood (i.e., nephropathy with continued illness since age 4), recurring parental separation, and perhaps also their guilt about his illness which progressively caused their final separation.

There were noticeable differences in the responses by Olivier and Jean-Michel at the time of their dialysis to the questionnaire about quality of life. Olivier experienced dialysis very negatively and seemed to deny anxiety about his illness, similar to many adolescents (Becker et al., 1979; Gutton, 1985). Jean-Michel accepted the passivity required for this long and repetitive treatment, and was able to continue constructive personal activity. He was further along in the adolescent process and regression was well accepted.

This conflict between passivity versus activity, and dependency versus independency is evident in their psychological assessments after transplantation, even though Olivier is now waiting again for a new transplant (but without registration on a list), and uncertainty is again stronger in that case for him (Weems and Patterson, 1989; Nekolaiuchuck, 1990; Juneau, 1995). With both patients, a rigid defensive system protects against the anxiety shown in the projective tests. The somatic anxiety is very much there with enormous body preoccupations. But there again Olivier and Jean-Michel differ in their mental functioning.

The suggested similarity between the adolescent process and the organ transplant process can be found in the protocols of

Olivier and Jean-Michel. The intricate relationship between castration anxiety and body image appears fundamental. Without a doubt, the actual experience and behavior of the transplanted adolescent who is confronted with the necessity of replacing a failing organ with somebody else's reactivates castration anxiety.

Olivier is similar to those adolescents observed on the Rorschach who present with an impairment of personality (Bourneuf and Bouras, 1980). Jean-Michel is not going through the adolescent process anymore, and the outcome of the reactivation of castration anxiety could depend more on the transplant process and his body's acceptance or rejection of the graft.

Olivier and Jean-Michel reacted differently to the "end of illness" that many patients associate with a kidney transplant. Olivier used an omnipotent defense and partial denial of his illness (our first hypothesis). The transplant had been idealized and any new frustration, such as therapeutic constraints related to the transplant, probably seemed intolerable to him. Such defenses and behavior are associated with noncompliance (Becker et al., 1979; Frazier et al., 1994).

But it is possible (and this is our second hypothesis) that the difficulty in attaining autonomy by the transplant patient is linked to marked dependency preceding adolescence, even if Olivier is presently unable to admit it. It seems that his dependency is linked to a defective internalization of a good-enough mother, making it difficult to be alone, and concurrently to a failure of paternal function.

Projective methods provided information on mental functioning, but a question remains. In such protocols, what can be imputed as a consequence of illness with an associated narcissistic wound? and what can be imputed to the adolescent developmental process which is incomplete, or earlier insults, and allows for narcissistic vulnerability? We suggest that, psychologically, a transplant implies recognition of a debt to the donor. This is similar to the adolescent development process which also involves acceptance of dependency on parents in earlier years. To attain independence the adolescent must be able to fit in with a family history which involves acceptance of past dependency and connection as part of identity. To be a self-sufficient, independent adult implies recognition of a sort of debt to one's parents. In the same way, the transplanted patient must find a satisfactory compromise between his personal autonomy and his dependency on the donor and the medical team. This gives him a different historical background for his identity. Olivier could not come to terms with this.

When a transplant occurs during adolescence many variables interfere. The reality of the illness is experienced as a narcissistic wound leading to a state of dependency, and is often felt by the child, and then the adolescent, as a real and symbolic castration (Crombez and Lefebvre, 1973). This is particularly so when the illness is discovered at an early age (Birraux, 1990), as in the case with Olivier. Did this contribute to some extent to his parents' gradual separation, and the destabilized parent–child relationship? In reverse, it would also seem evident that if the parents had been able to overcome their narcissistic wound in response to their child's and the future adolescent's illness, this would have contributed to the adolescent developmental process which integrates the physical deficit more harmoniously, and later enables integration of the graft. The self-esteem of a child or adolescent is dependent on the image that has been reflected to them by their parents' interest in their desires and successes, of their ability to admit and accept their failures, and finally the parents' support for the adolescents' future.

With a handicap such as ESRD, there can be compensation for, but not erasure of, the narcissistic wound. The adolescent is obliged to renounce any claim to a "perfect" body (Consoli and Bedrossian, 1979; Birraux, 1990). We hypothesize that narcissistic restoration could be possible with good maternal function, "a good-enough mother," in spite of the child's failures. On the other hand, the acceptance of a foreign graft as a part of the body (with respect to antirejection treatment) could be possible with proper paternal function, that is, integration of the inevitable castration feelings. The interrelation between internal and external reality at this particular moment in adolescence can either be a help, or on the contrary, reinforce the patient's handicap and difficulties.

It happens that at this point, Jean-Michel seemed to have a more detached and dynamic psychological functioning which enabled him to cope better with his state of ill-health. For Olivier, many important and unresolved problems seemed to be the cause of his difficulty in taking care of his transplant. His situation is perhaps more "uncertain" (Weems and Patterson, 1989; Nekolaiuchuck, 1990). Can we state that good emotional health determines better somatic functioning? Can we suppose that failure of kidney transplant occurs due to a patient's emotional difficulties? And, on the other hand, could a better state of physical health enable a patient to cope better?

CONCLUSION

From the literature review, it is generally believed and observed that compliance with therapy after end-stage renal disease and kidney transplant during adolescence is more difficult than any other time. This particular developmental stage already threatens the narcissistic status, and adolescents are considered to be predisposed to noncompliance because of their age more than any other factor. Uncertainty due to illness and waiting for a graft increases vulnerability. Two cases illustrate the general observations, and particularly the important influence of denial, depression, and anxiety on poor compliance. It is important for the adolescent to find a symbolic meaning in his or her illness after which a new identity, which integrates the illness, may emerge progressively based on narcissistic restoration.

Mental functioning, integration of the oedipal complex, and narcissistic status, also seem to play a part in compliance. Research with a sufficient number of subjects could allow us to define and detect psychological indicators of poor compliance. A systematic psychological follow-up of the vulnerable patients may avoid a part of these difficulties.

REFERENCES

Basch, S. H. (1973), The intrapsychic integration of a new organ. A clinical study of kidney transplantation. *Psychoanal. Quart.,* 42:364–384.

Baudin, M. (1989), Changer de coeur, continuer sa vie (Changing one's heart, continuing one's life). *Rev. Med. Psychosom.,* 30:87–101.

Becker, D., Igoin, L., & Delons, S. (1979), L'adolescent devant l'hémodialyse et la transplantation: Problèmes psychologiques et facteurs d'évolution (The adolescent confronted with dialysis and transplant: Psychological problems and developmental factors). *Arch. Franç. Pédiat.,* 36:313–319.

Birraux, A. (1990), *L'adolescent face à son corps. Emergences* (The adolescent confronted with his body. Emergence). Paris: Editions Universitaires.

Bourneuf, H., & Bouras, M. (1980), Le devenir psychologique des enfants transplantés rénaux (The psychological development of children with kidney transplants). *Neuropsychiatr. Enfance Adol.,* 28:555–563.

Brelet, F. (1986), *Le T.A.T., fantasme et situation projective* (The T.A.T. fantasy and projection). Paris: Dunod.

Bremer, B. A., Haffly, D., Foxx, R. M., & Weaver, A. (1995), Patients' perceived control over their health care: An outcome assessment of their psychological adjustment to renal failure. *Amer. J. Med. Qual.,* 10:149–154.

Calland, C. H. (1972), Iatrogenic problems in chronic renal disease. *New Eng. J. Med.,* 17:334–336.

Castelnuovo-Tedesco, P. (1973), Organ transplant, body images, psychosis. *Psychoanal. Quart.,* 42:349–363.

Chabert, C. (1983), Modalités du fonctionnement psychique des adolescents à travers le Roschach et le T.A.T. (Psychic functioning of adolescents who have undergone Rorschach and T.A.T. testing). *Psych. Franç.,* 28:187–194.

——— (1991), Interprétation des épreuves projectives à l'adolescence. Editions techniques (Interpretation of projective testing during adolescence). *Encyl. Med. Chir.* (Psychiatrie) 37213 B.

Chantler, X., Carter, J. E., Bewick, M., Counagan, R., Cameron, T. S., Ogg, C. S., Williams, D. G., & Winder, E. (1980), 10 years experience with regular heamodialysis and renal transplantation. *Arch. Dis. Child,* 55:435–445.

Christensen, A. J., Turner, C. W., Smith, T. W., Holman, J. M., & Gregory, M. C. (1991), Health locus of control and depression in end-stage renal disease. *J. Consult. Clin. Psychol.,* 59:419–424.

Consoli, S. M., & Bedrossian, J. (1979), Remaniements psychiques secondaires à une transplantation rénale (Psychic changes secondary to a kidney transplant). *Rev. Med. Psychosom.,* 3:299–307.

Crombez, J., & Lefebvre, P. (1973), La fantasmatique des greffés rénaux (Fantasies surrounding kidney grafts). *Rev. Fr. Psychanal.*, 37:95–107.

Douville, O. (1987), Le T.A.T. à l'adolescence (The T.A.T. and adolescence). *Psych. Franç.*, 32:161–167.

Ettenger, R. B., Rosenthal, J. T., Marik, J. L., Malekzadeh, M., Forsythe, S. B., Kamil, E. S., Salusky, I. B., & Fine, R. N. (1991), Improved cadaveric renal transplantation outcome in children. *Pediatr. Nephrol.*, 5:137–142.

Frazier, P. A., Davis-Ali, P. H., & Dahl, K. E. (1994), Correlates of noncompliance among renal transplant recipients. *Clin. Transplant.*, 8:550–557.

Gutton, P. (1985), La maladie, tache aveugle in corps souffrant (The illness, a blind spot in bodily suffering). *Adolescence*, 3:177–225.

Henning, P., Tomlinson, L., Rigden, S. P., Haycock, G. B., & Chantler, C. (1988), Long-term outcome of treatment of end-stage renal failure. *Arch. Dis. Child.*, 63:35–40.

Juneau, B. (1995), Psychologic and psychosocial aspects of renal transplantation. *Crit. Care Nurs. Quart.*, 17:62–66.

Kahn, A. U., Herndon, C. N., & Ahmadian, S. Y. (1971), Social and emotional adaptation of children with transplant kidneys and chronic hemodialysis. *Amer. J. Psychiatr.*, 127:114.

Kiley, D. J., Lam, C. S., & Pollack, R. (1993), A study of treatment compliance following kidney transplantation. *Transplantation*, 55:51–56.

Korsch, B. M., Fine, R., & Negrete, V. F. (1978), Noncompliance in children with renal transplant. *Pediatrics*, 61:872–876.

——— Negrete, V. F., Gardner, J. E., Weinstock, C. L., Mercer, A., Grushkin, C., & Fine, R. N. (1973), Kidney transplantation in children: Psychosocial follow-up study on child and family. *J. Pediatr.*, 13:399–408.

Leon, E., Baudin, M. L., & Consoli, S. M. (1990), Aspects psychiatriques des greffes d'organe. (Psychiatric aspects of organ grafts). Editions Techniques. *Encyl. Med. Chir.* (Psychiatrie), 37670 A65.

Levenson, H. (1973), Multidimensional locus of control in psychiatric patients. *J. Consult. Clin. Psychol.*, 41:397–404.

Litt, I. F., & Chriskey, W. R. (1980), Compliance with medical regimens during adolescence. *Pediatr. Clin. North Amer.*, 27:3–15.

Malekzadeh, M., Pennisi, A. J., Vittenbogaat, C. H., Korsch, B. M., Fine, R. N., & Main, M. E. (1976), Current issues in pediatric renal transplantation. *Pediatr. Clin. North Amer.*, 23:857–872.

Melzer, S. M., Leadbeater, B., Reisman, L., Jaffe, L. R., & Lieberman, K. V. (1989), Characteristics of social networks in adolescents with end-stage renal disease treated with renal transplantation. *J. Adol. Health Care*, 10:308–312.

Morton, M. J., Reynolds, J. M., Garralda, M. E., Postlethwaite, R. J., & Goh, D. (1994), Psychiatric adjustment in end-stage renal disease: A follow-up study of former pediatric patients. *J. Psychosom. Res.*, 38:293–303.

Nekolaiuchuck, C. L. (1990), Learning to live with uncertainty: The role of hope and medication compliance in chronic illness. Unpublished master's thesis, University of Alberta, Edmonton, Canada.

Poznanski, E. O., Miller, E., Salguerro, C., & Kelsch, R. C. (1978), Quality of life for long-term survivors of end-stage renal disease. *J. Amer. Med. Assn.*, 239:2343–2347.

Raimbault, G. (1973), Psychological aspects of chronic renal failure and haemodialysis. *Nephron.*, 11:252–260.

Reynolds, J. M., Garralda, M. E., Postlethwaite, R. J., & Goh, D. (1991), Changes in psychosocial adjustment after renal transplantation. *Arch. Dis. Child.*, 66:508–513.

—— Morton, M. J., Garralda, M. E., Postlethwaite, R. J., & Goh, D. (1993), Psychosocial adjustment of adult survivors of a pediatric dialysis and transplant program. *Arch. Dis. Child.*, 68:104–110.

Shaben, T. R. (1993), Psychosocial issues in kidney-transplanted children and adolescents: Literature review. *Amer. Nephrology Nurses' Assn. J.*, 20:663–668.

Shentoub, V., Chabert, C., Azoulay, C., Bailly-Salin, M. J., Benfredj, K., Boekholt, M., Brelet-Foulard, F., Chretien, M., Emanuelli, M., Martin, M., Monin, E., Peruchon, M., & Serviere, A. (Groupe de recherches en psychologie projective, Université René Descartes, Paris) (1990), *Manuel d'utilisation du T.A.T. Approche psychanalytique* (T.A.T. Manual: A psychoanalytic approach). Paris: Dunod.

Slama, L. (1987), *L'adolescent et sa maladie—Etude psychopathologique de la maladie chronique à l'adolescence.* (The adolescent and his illness—A study of psychopathology during chronic illness in adolescents). CTNER. numéro hos série. Paris: Presses Universitaires de France.

Tisza, V. B., Dorsett, P., & Morse, J. (1976), Psychological implications of renal transplantation. *J. Acad. Child. Psych.*, 15:709–720.

Weems, J., & Patterson, E. T. (1989), Coping with uncertainty and ambivalence while awaiting a cadaveric renal transplant. *Amer. Nephrology Nurses' Assn. J.*, 16:27–31.

8

The Developmental Impact of Cancer Diagnosis and Treatment for Adolescents

Margaret L. Stuber, M.D., and Anne E. Kazak, Ph.D.

Chronic or life-threatening pediatric illness intensifies the challenge of the major developmental tasks of adolescence. Issues of autonomy, peer relations, and future orientation may be complicated by the dependency of the patient role, the social isolation that treatment often requires, and the potential uncertainty of chronic or relapsing conditions. One of the best studied examples is pediatric cancer. The prognosis for children diagnosed with acute lymphoblastic leukemia (ALL), the most common childhood malignancy, has dramatically improved over the past twenty years. Kellerman and Katz (1977, p. 127) commented that the life expectancy had improved from three months in 1940 to "periods of remission ranging into several years." Today the five-year survival for ALL is approximately 70 percent (Parker, Tong, Bolden, and Wingo, 1996). The clinical concern has therefore turned to the long-term impact on survivors.

This study was supported by the National Cancer Institute (R0-63930) to Dr. Kazak and the National Institute of Mental Health (K07-MH01604) to Dr. Stuber.

REVIEW OF THE LITERATURE

A number of investigators have studied the psychological impact of cancer diagnosis and treatment on pediatric survivors (Koocher and O'Malley, 1981; Fritz, Williams, and Amylon, 1988; Mulhern, Wasserman, Friedman, and Fairclough, 1989; Kazak and Meadows, 1989; Spirito, Stark, Cobiella, Drigan, Androkites, and Hewitt, 1990). Most of these studies have found that the majority of survivors are functioning well, and do not differ significantly from healthy controls in overall psychological adjustment, or in prevalence of anxiety or depression. Only a small subset appears to have serious problems. For example, the classic study by Koocher and O'Malley (1981) found that 53 percent of 117 survivors appeared to be well-adjusted, although 11 percent had severe to disabling problems, and problems with school, work, and peer relations were common. A telephone survey of ninety-five adult survivors of pediatric malignancy found them to be functioning normally in educational achievement, occupational status, interpersonal relationships, marital status, pregnancies, employee benefits and insurance, and medical and health behaviors (Meadows, McKee, and Kazak, 1989).

However, the cancer experience does appear to have some lasting effects on the majority of survivors. A survey of 271 childhood cancer survivors, aged 14 to 29, examined the ways in which these young people felt they had been changed by cancer and treatment. The vast majority (76%) indicated that they felt that they were different from their agemates because they had cancer. Of these, 69 percent indicated that the differences were positive, while 31 percent referred to negative differences. The most frequently mentioned difference was the feeling that they were more advanced or mature in their personality or psychological development than their peers. Eighteen percent felt they knew more about life and their purpose in life than their peers, which they viewed as positive. A negative, reported by 16 percent, was feeling less healthy and less physically able than their peers who had not had cancer (Chesler, Weigers, and Lawther, 1992).

Similar findings were reported from an interview study of sixty-six childhood cancer survivors ages 8 to 20 years. Changes in their bodies as a result of the cancer or treatment were endorsed by 42.4 percent of the survivors. In a more global question, 51.5 percent of the survivors described themselves as different as a result of the cancer experience. The vast majority (70 to 90%) described these differences as positive. These included improvements in the way they treat others and make friends, the way their family and others treat them, the quality of their schoolwork and behavior, as well as their plans for the future and thoughts about life (Kazak, Stuber, Barakat, and Meeske, 1996).

Thus it appears that concern about the impact on their bodies, both functional and cosmetic, is pervasive, despite other apparently positive effects of the cancer experience. The impact on body image was supported by a recent study of forty-two adolescent and young adult female survivors of pediatric leukemia (mean age = 18.6 years, SD = 3.9 years). Self-assessment, clinical psychiatric assessment, and Rorschach tests all found the body images of the cancer survivors to be significantly inferior to those of sixty-nine healthy age-matched controls (Puuko, Hirvonen, Aalberg, Hovi, Rautonen, and Siimes, 1997).

To some extent, these perceptions could be seen as reflections of the fact that there are a number of concrete medical sequelae of cancer treatment (Meister and Meadows, 1993). Survivors of childhood cancer are often shorter than their peers (Holmes, Holmes, Baker, and Hassanein, 1990), and are at risk for neuropsychiatric sequelae, such as learning deficits, as a result of chemotherapy and radiation (Eiser, 1991; Mulhern, Fairclough, and Ochs, 1991). However, the medical and cognitive sequelae seem generally independent of the emotional responses. Only learning impairments have been found to significantly correlate with psychological distress in adolescent cancer survivors (Kazak, Christakis, Alderfer, and Coiro, 1994).

The studies by Koocher and O'Malley (1981), Chesler et al. (1992), and Puuko et al. (1997) combined adolescent subjects with young adults. Kazak et al. (1996) combined younger children with adolescents. Such mixing of populations makes it difficult to know to what extent the developmental phase of the survivor has influenced the results. Even combining younger and older adolescents includes a broad range of development, with a variety of issues. Studies that have limited their subjects to adolescents generally have smaller samples, and more limited questions. These have more clearly defined the areas of the problems, as well as the unaffected areas. For example, a study of fifty-four adolescent cancer patients found trait anxiety and self-esteem scores similar to those of a healthy comparison group, although the oncology patients reported a more external locus of control for health and higher impact of illness than the healthy group (Zeltzer and LeBaron, 1985). Good or excellent global functioning was reported by 61 percent of forty-one adolescent cancer survivors, with self-concept higher than normative values. Sixty percent identified a positive effect of their illness. However, concerns about their bodies were reported by over half of the group (Fritz et al., 1988)

CANCER AS DEVELOPMENTAL CHALLENGE

The perception that they are different from their peers, even if the differences are seen as positive, could be isolating for adolescents with cancer, and problematic for development. The negative impact of poor self-image on cooperation with treatment was documented in a study of twenty-seven adolescent cancer patients (Jamison, Lewis, and Burish, 1986). Negative self-perception is not the only reason for the common problems with adolescents' relative lack of cooperation with, or adherence to, treatment (Cromer and Tarnowski, 1989). However, it may serve to further isolate adolescents who are on active treatment or recovering from cancer. Such self-imposed separation was evident among the participants in an experimental psychotherapy group for adolescent cancer patients (Stuber, Gonzalez, Benjamin, and Golant, 1995). Using the format developed by the Wellness Community, a national organization for adults with cancer, groups were held concurrently for adolescents and their mothers. Transcripts of the two groups showed that the adolescents used the group to talk about their experiences, but did very little of the mutual problem solving that occurred in the mothers' group, and is typical of groups of adult cancer patients. Prominent themes in the adolescent group were how little their parents understood them or their experience, how isolated they felt from peers, and their difficulty in imagining a time in the future that would be different for them. The isolation appeared to be at least partly self-imposed, as expressed in their belief that it would be "weird" for a peer to really want to come see them in the hospital. When the group was visited by young adults who were now long-term survivors of pediatric cancer, the adolescents were very interested in the current lives of the survivors, and appeared eager to hear of the "normality" they had achieved. However, the adolescents did not want any advice, and did not appear persuaded that they would see their experience differently in the future.

This experience with group psychotherapy for adolescent cancer patients is similar to that reported by Baider and De-Nour (1989). Half of the sixteen candidates for the group refused to join, and those who did come discussed only "normal adolescent concerns" such as peer relations, parents, and future studies, but not the cancer after an initial period of disclosure. This resistance of adolescents with cancer to participate in any sort of psychotherapy group may be a part of a distancing and avoidant defense, and is consistent with clinical observations of the reluctance of adolescents to speak about aspects of the cancer experience to others (Kellerman and Katz, 1977). Investigation of information preferences among sixty-three adolescent cancer patients found that patients under active treatment were less desirous of additional information. Younger adolescents wanted to get information only from their parents, avoided group discussion, and did not want friends to receive additional information (Levonson, Pfefferbaum, Copeland, and Silberberg, 1982). Knowledge of illness by the adolescent appears to be related to that of the adolescent's family (Susman, Hersh, Nannis, Strope, Woodruff, Pizzo, and Levine, 1982), although significant parent–adolescent disparities are noted in the relative importance of disease-related information items and cancer-related tests and treatments (Levonson,

Copeland, Morrow, Pfefferbaum, and Silberberg, 1983). Interviews with three childhood cancer survivors who had been identified as "resiliant" (defined as unusually good adaptation in the face of severe stress) found that all had detailed, in-depth memories of the illness and treatments. They believed that relationships were key to their adjustment, and that self-understanding and putting cancer into perspective were important (Beardslee, 1989).

Researchers have examined the issue of denial or avoidance from a variety of perspectives. Some have hypothesized that children with cancer use denial when confronted with direct questions concerning their emotional responses (Worchel, Rae, Olson, and Crowley, 1992). Others have seen it as a "repressive adaptation," with repression associated with fewer self-reported depressive symptoms (Canning, Canning, and Boyce, 1992). In a study of sixty-six childhood cancer patients compared to 414 healthy children, the cancer patients were more likely to use an avoidant coping style than the controls. The tendency to use avoidant coping or "blunting" (defined as avoiding threat-relevant information when under stress), was positively correlated with time since diagnosis (Phipps, Fairclough, and Mulhern, 1995). A study of 177 children and adolescents (ages 7 to 18 years) with varying chronic illness found that the only consistent difference between coping styles used by children and adolescents was that adolescents were likely to use resignation as a coping strategy more often than younger children. Coping strategies used for illness-related and common problems were similar (Spirito, Stark, and Gil, 1995). This was not seen with a sample of childhood cancer survivors, in remission after completing treatment, who demonstrated different coping strategies for cancer-related and noncancer-related stressors (Bull and Drotar, 1991).

CANCER AS TRAUMA

A relatively new perspective on the developmental impact of childhood cancer is the concept of the cancer diagnosis and treatment as traumatic, with a more intense impact with other stressful events. Early clinical observers noted that children's responses to life-threatening illness were similar to those of survivors of events which were recognized to be traumatic (Nir, 1985; Pot-Mees, 1989; Stuber, Nader, Yasuda, Pynoos, and Cohen, 1991). These included intrusive memories or thoughts about the experience, avoidance of reminders, blunting emotions or anxiety, hypervigilance, and increased physiologic arousal. However, the *Diagnostic and Statistical Manual* (DSM-III-R; APA, 1987) specifically listed chronic illness as an exclusion to making a diagnosis of posttraumatic stress disorder (PTSD). This diagnosis is unusual among psychiatric diagnoses in that the etiology of the illness is specified as a criteria for diagnosis. Chronic illness was not considered to be "outside the range of usual human experience," as were the rest of the events considered capable of provoking the symptoms of PTSD.

Based on data from field trials with adolescent cancer survivors and pediatric gastrointestinal patients and their mothers, the 1994 revision of DSM-IV altered the criteria for posttraumatic stress disorder, identifying life-threatening illness as a possible antecedent event (APA, 1994). Since then, a number of studies have documented the presence of symptoms of posttraumatic stress in cancer patients, during and after active treatment. In one study, 106 women were evaluated for evidence of intrusive and avoidant symptoms before and six weeks following surgery for breast cancer. Eighteen percent of the women reported high levels of intrusive symptoms, and 14 percent reported high levels of avoidance on the Impact of Event Scale (Tjemsland, Soreide, and Malt, 1996). Breast cancer patients who have successfully completed treatments have also reported substantial numbers of symptoms of posttraumatic stress (Cordova, Andrykowski, Kenady, McGrath, Sloane, and Redd, 1995; Koopman, Classen, Butler, Duran, and Spiegel, 1996) although not always in the proper constellation to meet criteria for a diagnosis of PTSD (Alter, Pelcovitz, Axelrod, Goldenberg, Harris, Meyers, Grobois, Mandel, Septimus, and Kaplan, 1996). Mothers of adolescent cancer survivors have also been noted to report symptoms of posttraumatic stress disorder (Pelcovitz, Goldenberg, Kaplan, and Weinblatt, 1996; Stuber, Christakis, Houskamp, Pynoos, and Kazak, 1996).

Studies of survivors of childhood cancer have shown that a subset of children and adolescents report symptoms of posttraumatic stress (Butler, Rizzi, and Handwerger, 1996; Stuber, Christakis, Houskamp, Pynoos, and Kazak, 1996). When 319 childhood cancer survivors, ages 8 to 20 years, and their parents were compared to 214 children without a significant medical history and their parents, mothers and fathers of survivors reported significantly more symptoms of posttraumatic stress than mothers and fathers of comparison children. However, although almost 15 percent of survivors reported moderate to severe posttraumatic stress symptoms related to the cancer and treatment experience, statistical evaluation showed no significant differences in severity of symptoms reported when these survivors were compared to healthy controls (Kazak, Barakat, Meeske, Christakis, Meadows, Casey, Panati, and Stuber, 1997; Barakat, Kazak, Meadows, Casey, Meeske, and Stuber, 1997).

The studies suggest that although symptoms of posttraumatic stress appear to decrease with time, persistent symptoms remain for many years in a subset of childhood cancer survivors. In addition to time since completing treatment, gender (girls report more symptoms than boys) and other stressful life events are also significant, objectively quantifiable predictors of persistent posttraumatic stress disorder symptoms in childhood cancer survivors more than one year after completing treatment. However, the other significant predictors are subjective factors. General anxiety and subjective appraisal of life threat and treatment intensity made significant independent contributions to the severity of posttraumatic symptoms. Treatment-related objective stressors, such as physician-rated intensity of the treatment protocol or severity of medical sequelae, were not significant, independent contributors to severity of symptoms. Mothers' perception of treatment and life threat contributed to anxiety and subjective appraisal for the survivor, but did not independently contribute to posttraumatic stress disorder symptoms (Stuber, Kazak, Meeske, Barakat, Guthrie, Garnier, Pynoos, and Meadows, 1997).

Of the subjects in the study described above, 194 were aged 13 to 20 years at the time they completed the Posttraumatic Stress Disorder Reaction Index, a 24-item screening instrument for PTSD (Frederick, Pynoos, and Nader, 1992). A summary of the symptoms reported by more than 10 percent of the adolescents is seen in Table 8.1.

TABLE 8.1

Items endorsed on the Posttraumatic Stress Reaction Index by more than 10 percent of 194 childhood cancer survivors 13 to 20 years old. All refer to responses to the cancer experience (both diagnosis and treatment).

	%
Cancer Is Upsetting to Most People	36.4
Think Differently about the Future	31.0
Changed Activities	22.8
Changed Way I Get Along with People	19.1
Increased Risk Taking	15.6
Increased Startle	14.6
Feel More Alone Inside	14.4
Sleep Well (reversed)	13.6
More Stomachaches, Headaches	12.0
Stay Away from Reminders	10.8
Afraid or Upset When Think About the Cancer	10.8

Since there are no norms on this measure for adolescents who have not been exposed to traumatic events, the results must be interpreted with caution. However, it is interesting to note that the symptoms most commonly endorsed reflect changes that might not be readily apparent to an observer, but that could have long-term developmental impact. When only those adolescent survivors who reported moderate to severe levels of symptoms were examined, the distribution looks more like what we might expect from someone who has been traumatized. Table 8.2 summarizes the symptoms reported by more than 30 percent of these 46 symptomatic adolescents.

Another study, involving interviews of ten adolescents who had bone marrow transplants (BMT) as part of their treatment for cancer, suggests one functional consequence of both the sense

TABLE 8.2

Items endorsed on the Posttraumatic Stress Reaction Index by more than 30 percent of 46 adolescents aged 13 to 20 years, with total Reaction Index scores of 25 or greater. All refer to changes noted in response to the cancer experience (both diagnosis and treatment).

	%
More Stomachaches, Headaches	83.0
Increased Risk taking	83.0
Changed Activities	77.0
Cancer is Upsetting to Most People	74.0
Afraid or Upset with Thoughts of Event	58.7
Increased Startle	52.2
Feel More Alone Inside	47.8
Think Differently about the Future	47.4
Changed Way I Get Along with Other People	40.9
Tense or Upset when Reminded	39.2
Intrusive Memories	39.2
Avoid Reminders	36.9
Reexperiencing Event	34.8
Fears	33.4
Sleep Problems	32.6
Numbing	30.5

of being different from peers and having been exposed to trauma. Since BMT involves a month or more of isolation and extremely intense treatment, and only approximately 50 percent of those who undergo BMT survive more than a year posttransplant, these adolescent BMT survivors had clearly been exposed to life threat and assaults on their body integrity. Despite this clear risk, none of the survivors reported symptoms of posttraumatic stress disorder in the moderate or severe range. However, the control group in this study, comprised of friends who had been selected by the subjects, reported more symptoms of posttraumatic stress in response to various events in their lives than the subjects. Events reported by the controls included physical injuries to themselves as well as illnesses of family members. This suggests that there may be a tendency of childhood cancer survivors to select friends who had also experienced events which would shape their perspectives and set them apart from others (Stuber and Nader, 1995).

Another perspective on this topic was raised by another recent study of childhood cancer survivors. Evaluation of self-reports from forty adolescents and young adults found a significant association between denial of distress and higher levels of intrusive memories and avoidance, which are symptoms of PTSD (Erikson, Kato, Ketner, and Steiner, 1996). Since the sample was not limited to adolescents, the developmental implications of this finding are not clear. However, it is consistent with the observations cited above regarding the inclination of cancer patients in general, and adolescents in particular, to use repressive coping or denial. It also raises interesting questions regarding the potential consequences of this coping style.

CASE ILLUSTRATIONS

Two cases may illustrate the experience and thinking of adolescents dealing with cancer. Both adolescents were interviewed as a part of the large study of childhood cancer survivors described above, using the Impact of Traumatic Stressors Interview Schedule (Kazak et al., 1996). These are representative of the types of statements made by the sample. The information regarding their situations has been changed to protect confidentiality. The statements made are taken verbatim from the interviews.

CASE 1

Joseph is a 17-year-old Hispanic male who was diagnosed and treated for lymphoma when he was 10, and just completing the fifth grade. He remembers feeling tired, trouble breathing, as well as losing his appetite. "I never thought it would be cancer." His parents told him that, "I stopped breathing so they had machines hooked up to me. I was supposed to take radiation but I didn't because my dad didn't want me to. He thought just chemotherapy was okay." His own memories are more visceral. "The smell of foods reminds me of what smells I smelt at the time I was getting chemotherapy. And how they made me sick. . . . It's like when I was getting chemotherapy and my mom would bring me tea and a cup of soup. And now I can't have those two together, or tea and toast, 'cause if I do, it reminds me of the times when I'd thrown it all up. And I can still taste it and smell it. There are certain foods I can't eat together. Mostly tea and toast." There are also more specific reminders. "Some people—nurses and doctors—remind me of spinal taps and like how many times I had to go through them and how much it hurt and what I had to go through after." He talks about the consequences of the illness for him. "Taking the chemo . . . I couldn't do things. It would make me sick, so I couldn't sit and watch TV. I couldn't talk to anybody . . . I just wanted to sleep. There wasn't anything that could make me not feel that way . . . I felt like life was going on without me." His concerns now are, "I just might not be able to have children. Or that I might get cancer again. Any kind of cancer just 'cause I fear it. Scared that my children might get it also—if I am able to have children." Yet, despite all these negative memories and future concerns, when asked about ways in which he is different now because of the cancer experience, his response is primarily positive. "I've been through more things than I would've before, so that has made me more mature. I understand. . . . I am more understanding with problems. I go through life a little more carefully than I would normally. I watch what I do, as in what I eat, and how I take care of my body, and I watch my brother and sister grow differently, and I also look at the Earth differently. I appreciate it more. . . . Some people treat me with more respect. They know that I've gone through something even an adult would have trouble going through."

CASE 2

Susan, a 20-year-old woman of European ancestry, was 16 when she was diagnosed with osteogenic sarcoma. When asked what she remembers, she says, "I remember a lot. I remember when I was first told I just like was so overwhelmed. I couldn't believe it.

They did a whole bunch of tests and the first thing they said was they thought that I had a tumor on my heart. That just floored me. I was like, oh my God, you know, and so they made all the arrangements for me to come down here and I went right in here into intensive care." She remembers the chemotherapy making her sick, and getting stretch marks on her hips from the prednisone. "So, and I remember that I had some friends that were friends but once I had the cancer I realized many of them weren't, and some of them I thought were just OK friends I realized were really good friends. So when it happened to us, it really made us turn our whole life around. Really, we thought a lot different, especially me, about life." Her worst moment was when her hair fell out. She states she was most frightened when she had a spinal tap and the "doctor in training, she tried once and couldn't do it . . . it just freaked me out." Many things continue to remind her of the experience. "My experience with cancer is always in my everyday life. There are all kinds of little things that remind me of it. . . . I guess I think about it pretty much every day. I mean, cancer made me realize how precious life is, and before I didn't realize that." She worries about the future, but does not see it as related to her cancer or treatment. "I don't know what I'm worried about might happen. I'm sure just with old age something's bound to happen." Susan feels that she is different now as a result of the cancer. "I'm a lot more mature than I would be and I look at life in a better perspective. I take life day by day instead of thinking way ahead, because I never know, nobody ever knows if they'll live 'til tomorrow."

Discussion

These two cases demonstrate the types of long-term consequences which are reported by adolescent survivors of childhood cancer. Both survivors report some symptoms of intrusive memories and avoidance, indicating that they have been traumatized by the experience, but do not experience the number and severity of symptoms warranting a diagnosis of posttraumatic stress disorder. They give clear evidence that they see themselves as substantially changed by the experience, and that it has altered their perspective of their lives. However, the changes they describe in their worldview are seen as positive. They do not appear to be globally repressing or denying their experience, but speak of the life threat, discomfort, and fear quite clearly. They report enough negative symptoms and memories to make it unlikely that they are simply making what they perceive to be the socially correct responses.

It is not clear from these interviews what specific aspect(s) of the cancer experience constitute the traumatic or life-changing event(s) for these two individuals. Although it is the life-threatening diagnosis that is cited in the DSM-IV as the traumatic antecedent to symptoms, other studies have suggested that aspects of treatment are experienced as the "worst moments" or are more difficult or frightening for some children (Stuber, Nader, Houskamp, and Pynoos, 1996). The chronic intrusive nature of many treatment protocols raises the issue of whether childhood cancer survivors' symptoms are at least partially in response to a series of traumatic episodes (Stuber, Christakis et al. 1996). Answering this question would aid in interventions geared at preventing the development, and maintenance, of traumatic stress symptoms. It might also assist in understanding the types of symptoms that would be expected, since there is some evidence that acute, single episode traumas have different consequences than repeated traumas (Terr, 1991).

Another unanswered question is the interaction between age at diagnosis, and how the diagnosis and treatment are experienced and interpreted by the survivor. There are some data suggesting that older childhood cancer patients may have a better understanding of the prognosis of their illness and are more responsive to life-threat, while younger patients are more responsive to acute pain during active treatment (Stuber and Nader, 1995; Stuber, Nader et al., 1996). However, it is not clear whether there is a critical period when the traumatic aspect of the cancer experience has more significant long-term consequences. Age at diagnosis was not a significant contributor to the variability in severity of posttraumatic stress disorder symptoms in the study of 320 childhood cancer survivors described above (Stuber et al., 1997). However, changes in worldview would be more likely during periods of character development, such as early childhood and adolescence. The potential for trauma to influence character development has been explored in the proposal of a diagnostic category for the DSM called Disorders of Extreme Stress Not Otherwise Specified (DESNOS). This diagnosis is conceptualized as a response to trauma involving difficulty in affect modulation, maintenance of interpersonal boundaries, and changes in worldview (van der Kolk, Pelcovitz, Roth, Mandel, McFarlane, and Hermann, 1996). Although this was not accepted as a diagnosis for inclusion in the DSM-IV, it remains a topic of investigation, and is consistent with the considerations discussed above.

If childhood cancer creates a relatively subtle change in the developmental trajectory, a question of interest is what impact the changes in body image and worldview have on the life-choices that are commonly made in young adulthood. Preliminary data from an ongoing study of young adults who had childhood cancer suggest that these survivors report more symptoms than younger survivors, similar to parents of survivors (Hobbie, Meeske, Stuber, Wissler, Ruccione, Hinkle, and Kazak, 1998). Thus, it may be that childhood cancer patients are traumatized by the experience, but they do not experience the typical constellation of symptoms until they reach adulthood. An alternative explanation is that denial leads to underreporting of symptoms in younger survivors. Further research is needed to clarify this point.

Acute stress disorder (ASD), a diagnostic category newly added to the DSM-IV, presents interesting possibilities for further studies. The symptoms of ASD are similar to those of PTSD except that (1) they are manifest in the first month following the traumatic event (PTSD criteria require a symptom duration of at least a month), and (2) symptoms must include dissociation. Dissociation in the acute posttrauma period has been found to be a major predictor of PTSD. A study of ASD in cancer patients found that 41 percent of their sample met criteria for the diagnosis (McGarvey and Canterbury, 1996). This is a topic that warrants further investigation.

It should be noted that these adolescents are living and growing within the context of a family, which helps to shape their experience. Mothers and fathers of childhood cancer survivors report clinically and statistically significant levels of posttraumatic stress symptoms (Kazak et al., 1997). It is not clear how this affects the perspective of the adolescent, although it appears to have some impact (Stuber, Meeske, Gonzalez, Houskamp, Pynoos, and Kazak, 1994; Stuber, Kazak et al., 1997).

CONCLUSION

It no longer seems adequate to ask the somewhat simplistic question, "Are there adverse psychiatric sequelae of childhood cancer for adolescents?" It is relatively clearly established that the majority of childhood cancer survivors do not report symptoms consistent with major psychiatric diagnoses, and are generally functioning well in school and the workplace. More interesting are the questions about the adaptations made by adolescents, and the consequences of using common coping styles such as denial or blunting. Are adolescent cancer survivors denying their emotional symptoms as well, perhaps even to themselves? Or is this coping style so effective that they are not getting depressed or anxious? What are the interpersonal consequences of the sense of difference they report? Do they choose to be with others with similar backgrounds or responses?

What appears to be true is that childhood cancer survivors see themselves as changed by the experience. One of the changes is a heightened sense of vulnerability, resulting in a perspective of valuing each day. The survivors see this as a positive change. Although a clinician might frame this response in terms of the vigilance of posttraumatic stress, the data suggest that this change in perspective is not a pathological response but represents an adaptive response of resilient individuals.

REFERENCES

Alter, C. L., Pelcovitz, D., Axelrod, A., Goldenberg, B., Harris, H., Meyers, B., Grobois, B., Mandel, F., Septimus, A., & Kaplan, S. (1996), Identification of PTSD in cancer survivors. *Psychosom.*, 37:137–143.

American Psychiatric Association (1987), *Diagnostic and Statistical Manual of Mental Disorders.* 3rd ed., rev. (DSM-III-R). Washington, DC: American Psychiatric Press.

———(1994), *Diagnostic and Statistical Manual of Mental Disorders*, 4th ed. (DSM-IV). Washington, DC: American Psychiatric Press.

Baider, L., & De-Nour, A. K. (1989), Group therapy with adolescent cancer patients. *J. Adol. Health Care*, 10:35–38.

Barakat, L., Kazak, A. E., Meadows, A., Casey, M., Meeske, K., & Stuber, M. L. (1997), Families surviving childhood cancer: A comparison of posttraumatic stress symptoms with families of healthy children. *J. Ped. Psychology*, 22(6):843–859.

Beardslee, W. R. (1989), The role of self-understanding in resilient individuals: The development of a perspective. *Amer. J. Orthopsychiatry*, 59:266–278.

Bull, B. A., & Drotar, D. (1991), Coping with cancer in remission: Stressors and strategies reported by children and adolescents. *J. Ped. Psychology*, 16:767–782.

Butler, R. W., Rizzi, L. P., & Handwerger, B. A. (1996), Brief report: The assessment of posttraumatic stress disorder in pediatric cancer patients and survivors. *J. Ped. Psychology*, 21:499–504

Canning, E. H., Canning, R. D., & Boyce, W. T. (1992), Depressive symptoms and adaptive style in children with cancer. *J. Amer. Acad. Child Adol. Psychiatry*, 31:1120–1124.

Chesler, M. A., Weigers, M., & Lawther, T. (1992), How am I different? Perspectives of childhood cancer survivors on changes and growth. In: *Late Effects of Treatment for Childhood Cancer*, ed. D. M. Green & G. J. D'Angio. New York: Wiley-Liss, pp. 151–158.

Cordova, M. J., Andrykowski, A., Kenady, D., McGrath, P. C., Sloane, D. A., & Redd, W. H. (1995), Frequency and correlates of post-traumatic stress disorder-like symptoms after treatment for breast cancer. *J. Cons. Clin. Psychology*, 63:981–986.

Cromer, B. A., & Tarnowski, K. J. (1989), Noncompliance in adolescents: A review. *Devel. Behav. Ped.*, 10:207–215.

Eiser, C. (1991), Cognitive deficits in children treated for leukemia. *Arch. Dis. Child.*, 55:164–168.

Erikson, S., Kato, P. M., Ketner, K., & Steiner, H. (1996), Denial of distress and posttraumatic stress symptomatology among long-term survivors of childhood cancer. Proceedings of the annual meeting of the International Society for Traumatic Stress Studies, San Francisco, November 10–13.

Frederick, C., Pynoos, R. S., & Nader, K. O. (1992), *The Posttraumatic Stress Reaction Index.* Typescript.

Fritz, G., Williams, J., & Amylon, M. (1988), After treatment ends: Psychosocial sequelae in pediatric cancer survivors. *Amer. J. Orthopsychiatry,* 58:552–561.

Hobbie, W., Meeske, K., Stuber, M., Wissler, K., Ruccione, K., Hinkle, A., & Kazak, A. (1998), Symptoms of posttraumatic stress in young adult survivors of childhood cancer. Young Adult Survivors of Childhood Cancer. Proceedings of the Fourth International Congress of Psycho-Oncology. Hamburg, Germany, September 3–6.

Holmes, G., Holmes, F. F., Baker, A. B., & Hassanein, R. S. (1990), Childhood cancer survivors: Attained adult heights compared with sibling controls. *Clin. Ped.,* 29:268–272.

Jamison, R. N., Lewis, S., & Burish, T. G. (1986), Cooperation with treatment in adolescent cancer patients. *J. Adol. Health Care,* 7:162–167.

Kazak, A. E., Barakat, L. P., Meeske, K., Christakis, D., Meadows, A. T., Casey, R., Panati, B., & Stuber, M. L. (1997), Posttraumatic stress symptoms, family functioning and social support in survivors of childhood leukemia and their mothers and fathers. *J. Clin. Cons. Psychology,* 65:120–129.

——— Christakis, D., Alderfer, M., & Coiro, M. J. (1994), Young adolescent cancer survivors and their parents: Adjustments, learning problems, and gender. *J. Fam. Psychology,* 8:74–84.

——— Meadows, A. (1989), Families of young adolescents who have survived cancer: Social–emotional adjustment, adaptability, and social support. *J. Ped. Psychology,* 14:175–191.

——— Stuber, M. L., Barakat, L. P., & Meeske, K. (1996), Assessing posttraumatic stress related to medical illness and treatment: The Impact of Traumatic Stressors Interview Schedule (ITSIS). *Fam., Syst. & Health,* 14:365–380.

——— ——— ——— ——— Casey, R., Penati, B., Guthrie, D., & Meadows, A. (in press), Predictors of posttraumatic stress symptoms in parents of childhood cancer survivors. *J. Amer. Acad. Child & Adoles. Psychiatry.*

Kellerman, J., & Katz, E. R. (1977), The adolescent with cancer: Theoretical, clinical, and research issues. *J. Ped. Psychology,* 2:127–131.

Koocher, G., & O'Malley, J. E. (1981), *The Damocles Syndrome: Psychosocial Consequences of Surviving Childhood Cancer.* New York: McGraw-Hill.

Koopman, C., Classen, C., Butler, L., Duran, R., & Spiegel, D. (1996), Factors associated with PTSD symptoms among primary breast cancer patients. Proceedings of the annual meeting of the International Society for Traumatic Stress Studies, San Francisco, November 10–12.

Levonson, P. M., Copeland, D. R., Morrow, J. R., Pfefferbaum, B., & Silberberg, Y. (1983), Disparities in disease-related perceptions of adolescent cancer patients and their parents. *J. Ped. Psychology,* 8:33–45.

——— Pfefferbaum, B., Copeland, D. R., & Silberberg, Y. (1982), Information preferences of cancer patients ages 11–20 years. *J. Adol. Health Care,* 3:9–13.

McGarvey, E. L., & Canterbury, R. J. (1996), Acute stress disorder in newly diagnosed cancer patients. Proceedings of the annual meeting of the International Society for Traumatic Stress Studies, San Francisco, November 10–12.

Meadows, A. T., McKee, L., & Kazak, A. E. (1989), Psychosocial status of young adult survivors of childhood cancer: A survey. *Med. Ped. Oncol.*, 17:466–470.

Meister, L., & Meadows, A. (1993), Late effects of childhood cancer therapy. *Curr. Prob. Ped.*, 23:102–131.

Mulhern, R., Fairclough, D., & Ochs, J. (1991), A prospective comparison of neuropsychologic performance of children surviving leukemia who receive 18Gy, 24Gy, or no cranial irradiation. *J. Clin. Oncol.*, 9:1348–1356.

―――― Wasserman, A., Friedman, A. G., & Fairclough, D. (1989), Social competence and behavioral adjustment of children who are long-term survivors of cancer. *Pediatrics*, 83:18–25.

Nir, Y. (1985), Posttraumatic stress disorder in children with cancer. In: *Posttraumatic Stress Disorder in Children*, ed. S. Eth & R. Pynoos. Washington, DC: American Psychiatric Press.

Parker, S. L., Tong, T., Bolden, S., & Wingo, P. A. (1996). Cancer statistics. *CA: Cancer J. for Clinicians*, 46:5–27.

Pelcovitz, D., Goldenberg, B., Kaplan, S., & Weinblatt, M. (1996), Post-traumatic Stress Disorder in mothers of pediatric cancer survivors. *Psychosom.*, 37:116–126.

Phipps, S., Fairclough, D., & Mulhern, R. K. (1995), Avoidant coping in children with cancer. *J. Ped. Psychology*, 20:217–232.

Pot-Mees, C. (1989), *The Psychosocial Effects of Bone Marrow Transplantation in Children*. Delft, Netherlands: Eubron Delft.

Puukko, L. M., Hirvonen, E., Aalberg, V., Hovi, L., Rautonen, J., & Siimes, M. A. (1997), Impaired body image of young female survivors of childhood leukemia. *Psychosom.*, 38:54–62.

Spirito, A., Stark, L., Cobiella, C., Drigan, R., Androkites, A., & Hewitt, K. (1990), Social adjustment of children successfully treated for cancer. *J. Ped. Psychology*, 15:359–371.

―――― ―――― Gil, K. M. (1995), Coping with everyday and disease-related stressors by chronically ill children and adolescents. *J. Amer. Acad. Child Adol. Psychiatry*, 34:283–290.

Stuber, M. L., Christakis, D., Houskamp, B. M., Pynoos, R. S., & Kazak, A. E. (1996), Post trauma symptoms in childhood leukemia survivors and their parents. *Psychosom.*, 37:254–261.

―――― Gonzalez, S., Benjamin, H., & Golant, M. (1995), Fighting for recovery: Group interventions for adolescents with cancer and their parents. *J. Psychother. Prac. Res.*, 4:286–296.

―――― Kazak, A. E., Meeske, K., Barakat, L., Guthrie, D., Garnier, H., Pynoos, R. S., & Meadows, A. (1997), Predictors of posttraumatic stress symptoms in childhood cancer survivors. *Pediatrics*, 100(6):958–964.

―――― Meeske, K., Gonzalez, S., Houskamp, B., Pynoos, R. S., & Kazak, A. (1994), Posttraumatic stress after childhood cancer I: The role of appraisal. *PsychoOnc.*, 3:303–312.

―――― Nader, K. O. (1995), Psychiatric sequelae in adolescent bone marrow transplantation survivors. *J. Psychother. Prac. Res.*, 4:30–32.

―――― ――――Houskamp, B. M., & Pynoos, R. S. (1996), Appraisal of life threat and acute trauma responses in pediatric bone marrow transplant patients. *J. Traum. Stress*, 9:673–686.

—— Nader, K., Yasuda, P., Pynoos, R. S., & Cohen, S. (1991), Stress responses following pediatric bone marrow transplantation: Preliminary results of a prospective, longitudinal study. *J. Amer. Acad. Child Adol. Psychiatry,* 30:952–957.

Susman, E. J., Hersh, S. P., Nannis, E. D., Strope, B. E., Woodruff, P. J., Pizzo, P. A., & Levine, A. S. (1982), Conceptions of cancer: The perspectives of child and adolescent patients and their families. *J. Ped. Psychology,* 7:253–261.

Terr, L. (1991), Childhood traumas: An outline and overview. *Amer. J. Psychiatry,* 148:10–20.

Tjemsland, L., Soreide, J. A., & Malt, U. F. (1996), Traumatic distress symptoms in early breast cancer II: Outcome six weeks post surgery. *PsychoOnc.,* 5:295–303.

van der Kolk, B., Pelcovitz, D., Roth, S., Mandel, F. S., McFarlane, A., & Herman, J. L. (1996), Dissociation, somatization and affect dysregulation: The complexty of adaptation to trauma. *Amer. J. Psychiatry,* 53 (suppl.; festschrift):83–93.

Worchel, F. F., Rae, W. A., Olson, T. K., & Crowley, S. L. (1992), Selective responses of chronically ill children to assessment of depression. *J. Person. Assess.,* 59:605–615.

Zeltzer, L., & LeBaron, S. (1985), Does ethnicity constitute a risk factor for the psychological distress of adolescents with cancer? *J. Adol. Health Care,* 6:8–11.

Part III

Social Disruption
and the Adolescent Process

9

What Children Can Tell Us about Living with Violence

JAMES GARBARINO, Ph.D.

Since security is vitally important for a child's well-being, when infants and children feel safe, they relax. When relaxed, they start to explore the environment. When a parent or other familiar person is around, a child treats the adult as a secure base from which to explore the nearby space. If frightened—perhaps by a loud sound or by the approach of a stranger—the child quickly retreats to the familiar person.

This pattern is part of the normal development of children. It is so common that it is used to assess the quality of children's attachment relations. Children who do *not* use their parents this way—showing anxiety when separated and relief when re-united—are thought to have a less than adequate attachment relationship (they are "insecure" or "ambivalent" or "avoid-ant"). Thus, for very young children, the question of security is relatively simple. As a parent, I remember clearly the physical experience of the clinging, wary child regarding a stranger. And I remember sitting in airports, or visiting friends, and serving as a secure base for a tiny explorer.

Of course as children get older, their security needs are trans-formed. Soon they are getting on school buses and visiting friends' houses by themselves. Eventually they are on the streets

165

at night on their own. But security remains a constant theme for them. Am I safe here? Will I be safe if I go there? Would I be safe then? Many children do not feel safe, and in some cases, their insecurity is grounded in fact. This paper explores exposure to community violence as a threat to children's well-being and mental health.

THE AMERICAN WAR ZONE

Violence is a fact of life for millions of American children. Television infuses imagery of violence into virtually every household; "real life" violence on the streets, in the schools, or in the form of child or spouse abuse touches millions directly. What do we know about the impact of all this violence on children and their development? What can children tell us about the meaning of violence in their lives?

Homicide rates provide only an imprecise indicator of the overall problem of violence in the lives of American children and youth, for behind each murder stand many nonlethal assaults. This ratio varies as a function of both medical trauma technology (which prevents assaults from becoming homicides) and weapons technology (which can increase or decrease the lethality of assaults). An example from Chicago illustrates this. The city's homicide rates in 1973 and 1993 were approximately the same, and yet the rate of serious assault increased approximately 400 percent during that period. Thus, the ratio of assaults to homicides increased substantially—from 1:100 in 1973 to 1:400 in 1993 (Garbarino, Dubrow, Kostelny, and Pardo, 1992).

Data from Chicago's Cook County Hospital provide another perspective on the changing nature of violence facing children in America. In 1982, the hospital responded to approximately 500 gunshot cases. In 1992, the number was approximately 1000. However, in 1982 almost all these cases involved single bullet injuries, while in 1992, 25 percent involved multiple bullets. Rates of permanent disability have thus increased substantially, although the homicide rate has shown only a modest increase.

Class, race, and gender exert important influences on exposure to community violence. The odds of being a homicide victim range from 1:21 for black males, to 1:369 for white females—with white males at 1:131, and black females at 1:104 (Bell, 1991). Being an American itself is a risk factor. The United States far exceeds all other modern industrialized nations in its homicide rate (even for whites, where the rate of 11.2 per 100,000 is far more than the second place country, Scotland, with 5 per 100,000 [Richters and Martinez, 1993]).

Whatever the exact constellation of causes, children growing up in the United States have particularly high levels of exposure to violence, especially if they live in neighborhoods that constitute "war zones." A survey of 6th to 10th graders in New Haven, Connecticut, revealed that 40 percent had witnessed at least one incident of violent crime within the last twelve months (Marans and Cohen, 1993). In three high risk neighborhoods in Chicago, 17 percent of the elementary school age children had witnessed domestic violence; 31 percent had seen someone shot; and, 84 percent had seen someone "beat up" (Bell, 1991). Some 30 percent of youngsters living in high crime neighborhoods of the large cities, such as Chicago, have witnessed a homicide by the time they are 15 years old, and more than 70 percent have witnessed a serious assault. These figures are much more similar to the experience of youngsters in the war zones we have visited in other countries (Garbarino, Kostelny, and Dubrow, 1991) than they are of what we should expect for our own children, living in "peace." Richters and Martinez (1993) have amplified these results. In their study, 43 percent of the 5th and 6th graders had witnessed a mugging in a *"moderately* violent" neighborhood in Washington, DC. Other researchers echo these findings (e.g., Groves, Zuckerman, Marans, and Cohen, 1993). Guns are one of the recurrent themes in the American war zone.

LIFE IS SCARY

Researchers working in inner-city high-crime neighborhoods report that by age 15 more than a third of the children have witnessed a homicide. A 6-year-old girl once told me that her job was to find her 2-year-old sister whenever the shooting started, and get her to safety in the bathtub of their apartment. "The bathroom is the safest place," she told me. Being responsible for the safety of another, younger child is too big a responsibility for a 6-year-old.

But this is not the whole story. For some children, the basis for their sense of insecurity is not life in the urban war zone, but just life. A national survey conducted by *Newsweek* and the Children's Defense Fund *(Newsweek,* 1992), found that only a minority of children, nationwide, said they felt "very safe" once they walked out the door. Most said they only felt "somewhat safe," and about 12 percent said they felt "unsafe." Other surveys report similar results. For example, a Harris poll of 6th to 12th graders several years ago revealed that 35 percent worried they would not live to old age because they would be shot (Harris and Associates, 1994). Why are even children in small towns and suburbs afraid? Why are even economically secure children afraid?

More and more children in the United States are experiencing a growing sense of insecurity about the world inside and outside the boundaries of their families. For one thing, they are preoccupied with kidnapping. Teacher after teacher in schools around the country tells me that if he or she asks students what they worry about, kidnapping looms large for most. One study reported that 43 percent of the elementary school children studied thought it was likely that they would be kidnapped (Price and Desmond, 1987). Having been bombarded with messages of threats via the news, and more informal sources (such as worried parents and other well-meaning adults), children have drawn the logical conclusion: if the adults are so scared, I should be too.

Being a child becomes more and more dangerous as chronic violence becomes a fact of life for more and more Americans.

Drugs, guns, and gangs conspire to create extremely dangerous environments for children and youth in urban neighbor-hoods—and increasingly, elsewhere in our society. These violent external threats often are added to the risk of violence inside the family, and the broader range of risk factors that afflict children in America (i.e., poverty, parental substance abuse, absent fathers, and maternal incapacity). These are risk factors that produce a "socially toxic" environment for children (Garbarino, 1995). These are the children of greatest concern to us, the children who face major accumulations of risk factors, and who are thus most at risk for the psychological effects of trauma due to vio-lence. These are children in danger.

In our interviews with families living in public housing projects in Chicago we learned that virtually all the children had first-hand experiences of shooting by the time they were 5 years old (Dubrow and Garbarino, 1989). Interviews with school-age chil-dren confirm that the "gun culture" is a potent factor in the lives of children in diverse settings in the United States (Garbarino, 1995). The spread of the "gun culture" into the lives of school-children is associated with a clear and present danger to their mental health, social behavior, and educational success. We base this conclusion upon an analysis of the role of trauma, threat, and violence on the development of children (Garbarino et al., 1992).

Perhaps a few examples will help illuminate the effects of this gun culture on the experience of childhood. In Detroit, a young boy whose idolized teenage brother was killed in a gang-related attack, was asked, "If you could have anything in the whole world, what would it be?" His answer: "A gun so I could blow away the person that killed my brother" (Marin, 1989). In California, when we asked a 9-year-old boy living in a neighborhood characterized by declining security, "What would it take to make you feel safer here?" he replied simply, "If I had a gun of my own" (Garbarino, 1995). In a middle-class suburb of Chicago, when we asked a classroom of 8-year-olds, "If you needed a gun could you get one?" a third of the children were able to describe in detail how they would get one. In a prison in North Carolina (Garbarino, 1995), when we asked three incarcerated teenagers about why they had done the shooting that had landed them in prison, all three replied, "What else was I supposed to do?"

We must understand the gun culture infusing the minds and hearts of American children and youth. Whether or not this cultural infusion results in actual shooting depends upon the particular circumstances of those children and youth; specifically, whether they experience an accumulation of social and psychological risk factors in the absence of compensatory opportunity factors.

THE CONSEQUENCES OF LIVING IN DANGER

One result of violence is psychological trauma for victims, particularly children. Coping with the consequences of escalating community violence has become a major focus of our national agenda (Garbarino et al., 1992). The emergent field of traumatic stress studies is increasingly recognizing the importance of understanding the phenomenon of posttraumatic stress disorder (PTSD) as a response to childhood trauma. This follows upon the inclusion of PTSD as a category for official diagnosis by the American Psychiatric Association. Diagnostic criteria for PTSD include reexperiencing the trauma (e.g., through recurrent dreams), numbing of responsiveness in day-to-day life, and a pattern of distorted feelings related to the traumatic experience such as feeling guilty about having survived while others did not (American Psychiatric Association, 1994).

What is only beginning to become clear is what happens to children when the dangers they face are not distinct and single events, but rather become the fabric of their lives. This is the distinction between *acute* danger (e.g., when a deranged individual enters a normally safe school and opens fire with a rifle) and *chronic* danger (e.g., when ongoing gang warfare makes a child's streets and school a battleground in which even "innocent bystanders" are in jeopardy).

Acute danger requires a process of adjustment, either through changing the conditions of life or changing one's stance toward life events. Acute incidents of danger often simply require *situational* adjustment by normal children leading normal lives—fitting the traumatic event into the child's understanding of his or her situation. The therapy of choice is reassurance: "You are safe again; things are back to normal."

This is not to deny that PTSD in children and youth exposed to acute danger may require processing over a period of months. If the trauma is intense enough, it may leave permanent psychic scars, particularly for children made vulnerable because of disruptions in their primary relationships (most notably with parents). These effects include excessive sensitivity to stimuli associated with the trauma and diminished expectations for the future.

CHRONIC DANGER AND ITS CONSEQUENCES FOR DEVELOPMENT

But what if there is no "post" trauma, and instead there is continuing exposure to trauma? Chronic danger imposes a requirement for *developmental* adjustment. Children may appear to "get used to it," but chronic danger is likely to produce far-reaching effects upon the child. These include chronic PTSD, alterations of personality, and major changes in patterns of behavior and beliefs to make some sense of ongoing danger. When these assaults occur in the context of a family or community experience that results in the child feeling ashamed of his or her identity, the possibilities for rage and further aggression increase.

Future orientation is important for children, and particularly adolescents, to attend to adult agendas for socialization. Trauma undermines future orientation. Some observers have identified a pattern of "terminal thinking" that affects those most affected. Terminal thinking is most clearly evident when, in response to the question, "What do you expect to be when you are 30 years old?'' the youth answers, "Dead." This outcome is most likely to take place when danger comes from social factors that overthrow day-to-day social reality, as happens during war, or when a child's neighborhood is taken over by chronic, violent crime.

The therapy of choice in situations of chronic danger is one which builds upon the child's primary relationships. The goal is to create a new positive reality for the child. This new reality must be able to stand up to the "natural" conclusions that a severely traumatized child is likely to draw otherwise: "I'm weak and worthless," "You can't rely upon adults," and, "The only way to be safe is to escape, or to get them before they get you."

Adolescent males (i.e., the "soldiers") are the predominant casualties of neighborhoods saturated with crime, particularly gang- and drug-related crime. For the most part, children are still "innocent bystanders" or "in training" for the front lines of violent conflict. Even when few children are actually shot, the process of adapting to the threat of violence can shape their development in many, mostly negative ways.

As noted earlier, surveys of youth on the southside of Chicago reveal that 25 percent of them have witnessed a murder by the time they were 17. Studies in other American cities such as Washington, DC, have confirmed and extended these findings. In our study of safety issues for children in public housing projects in Chicago, which are saturated with violence, mothers identify "shooting" as their major safety concern for their children. All the children have had first-hand experiences with shooting by age 5. Children, youth, and parents learn to adapt to living this way. *And that adaptation is part of the problem we face* (Garbarino et al., 1992).

THE ACCUMULATION OF RISK

Risk accumulates. This is one of the conclusions that we draw from our observations of children coping with chronic violence in today's America. Children are capable of coping with one or two major risk factors in their lives. But when risk accumulates—the addition of a third, fourth, and fifth risk factor—we see a precipitation of developmental damage (Sameroff, Seifer, Barocas, Zax, and Greenspan, 1987). This developmental model is particularly relevant to understanding the impact of chronic community violence on inner city children (Garbarino and Associates, 1992).

The experience of community violence takes place within a larger context of risk for most children. They often are poor, live in father-absent families, contend with parental incapacity due to depression or substance abuse, are raised by parents with little education or employment prospects, and are exposed to domestic violence (Kotlowitz, 1991).

This constellation of risk by itself creates enormous challenges for young children. For them, the trauma of community violence is often literally "the straw that breaks the camel's back." Bearing in mind that approximately 20 percent of American children live with this sort of accumulation of risk, the problem of violence is clearly a national problem with far-reaching implications for child development (Osofsky, 1995).

The task of dealing with the effects of this environmental conspiracy falls to the people who care for these children—their parents and other relatives, teachers, and counselors. But these adults who take on this task are facing enormous challenges of their own. We have found that human service professionals and educators working in the high violence areas of our communities are themselves traumatized by their exposure to violence (Garbarino et al., 1992).

In one study we found that 60 percent of the Head Start staff members surveyed in Chicago had experienced traumatic events connected with violence (Garbarino et al., 1992). For these individuals, their efforts to create a "safe zone" in the school are crucial to their ability to perform their important functions in the lives of high-risk children. For this safe zone to help children focus on their schoolwork, it must exist as part of their social maps.

THE SOCIAL MAPS OF CHILDREN IN DANGER

Certainly one of the most important features of child development is the child's emerging capacity to form and maintain "social maps" (Garbarino and Associates, 1992; Garbarino, 1995).
These representations of the world reflect the simple cognitive
competence of the child (knowing the world in the scientific
sense of objective, empirical fact), to be sure, but they also indicate the child's moral and affective inclinations.

We are concerned with the conclusions about the world contained in the child's social maps: "adults are to be trusted because
they know what they are doing"; "people will generally treat you
well and meet your needs"; "strangers are dangerous"; "school
is a safe place." The forces shaping these maps include the child's
experiences in counterpoint with the child's inner life—both the
cognitive competence and the working of unconscious forces.

Young children must contend with dangers that derive from
two sources which are not nearly so relevant to adults. First, their
physical immaturity places them at risk for injury from trauma
that would not hurt adults because they are larger and more
powerful. Second, young children tend to believe in the reality
of threats from what most adults would define as "the fantasy"
world. This increases their vulnerability to perceiving themselves
as being "in danger." These dangers include monsters under the
bed, wolves in the basement, and invisible creatures that lurk in
the dark corners of the bedrooms.

Trauma arises when the child cannot give meaning to dangerous experiences. This orientation is contained in the American
Psychiatric Association's (1994) definition of posttraumatic stress
disorder, which refers to life-threatening experiences. Herman
(1992) defined trauma thus: to come face-to-face with both human vulnerability in the natural world and with the capacity for
evil in human nature.

This suggests that trying to "understand" these experiences
may itself have pathogenic side effects. That is, in coping with
traumatic events, the child is forced into patterns of behavior,

thought, and feelings that are themselves "abnormal" when contrasted with that of the untraumatized healthy child. Children are particularly vulnerable to the trauma caused by threat and fear. Those exposed to trauma before age 10 were three times more likely to exhibit PTSD than those exposed after age 12 (Davidson and Smith, 1990).

Children who learn to live with chronic danger due to violence do not escape unscathed. Indeed, children forced to cope with chronic danger may adapt in ways that are dysfunctional. Children exposed to the stress of extreme violence (such as was the case in Cambodia) may reveal mental health disturbances years after the immediate experience is over. For example, a follow-up study of Cambodian children who experienced the moral and psychological devastation of the Pol Pot regime in the period 1974 to 1979 revealed that four years after leaving Cambodia 50 percent developed posttraumatic stress disorder (Kinzie, Sack, Angell, Manson, and Rath, 1986).

Children (and parents) may cope with danger by adopting a worldview that may be dysfunctional in "normal" situations in which they are expected to participate (e.g., in school). For example, their adaptive behavior in the abnormal situation of chronic crisis may be maladaptive to school success if they defend themselves by becoming hyperaggressive (which stimulates rejection at school). Such an adaptation may become a stable feature of personality and social ideology early in life. By age 8 patterns of aggressive behavior and "legitimization of aggression" tend to become stable, with predictability to adulthood (American Psychological Association, 1993).

Further, some adaptations to chronic danger, such as emotional withdrawal, may be socially adaptive in the short run, but become a danger to the next generation, when the individual becomes a parent. This phenomenon has been observed in studies of some families of Holocaust survivors. The emotional numbing that initially helped them to cope with life in the camps, put them at risk in the long run for emotional neglect of their own children (Danieli, 1988).

Parental adaptation to dangerous environments may produce child-rearing strategies that impede normal development. For example, the parent who prohibits the child from playing outside for fear of shooting incidents, may be denying the child a chance to engage in exploratory play, as an undesirable side effect of protecting the child from assault.

Similarly, the fear felt by parents of children in high crime environments may show up as a very restrictive and punitive style of discipline (including physical assault). The parent may see it as an effort to protect the child from falling under the influence of negative forces in the neighborhood (e.g., gangs). Unfortunately, this approach is likely to have the result of heightening aggression in the child. One consequence may be difficulty in succeeding in school and other contexts that provide alternatives to the gang culture.

Another possible adapation may be accepting violence as the modus operandi for social control (which in turn rationalizes the gang's use of violence as the dominant tactic for social influence). Holding the child back from negative forces through punitive restrictiveness is generally much less successful as a strategy than dealing with emotions openly, and promoting positive alternatives to the negative subculture feared by the parent. While understandable in the short run, such parental reliance on assault may be problematic in the long run.

In all of these examples, the adaptation is well-intentioned and may appear to be sensible and practical. It may even succeed in the immediate context as a kind of "psychosocial chemotherapy" that uses a poison in a desperate situation, and at great cost, to preserve the child in the midst of the crisis of a life-threatening social environment. But its side effects may be detrimental in the long run. The problem, of course, is the social forces that create and sustain danger in the family's environment.

Beyond the direct effects of parents, the children may be involved in the process of identification with the aggressor, in which they seek to emulate those powerful aggressive individuals and groups in their environment which cause the danger in the first place (e.g., gangs in the public housing project, or enemy soldiers under conditions of wartime occupation). "If you can't beat 'em, join 'em," seems a sensible strategy for many children. As a result, hundreds of thousands of American youth routinely carry weapons to school or in their neighborhoods. It makes them *feel* safer (even if the fact of the matter is that they are more likely to be involved in a lethal confrontation as a result).

One of our major concerns is that living in chronic danger will have a negative effect on the process of moral development. One result is likely to be the sort of "vendetta mentality" and "truncated" moral reasoning found among terrorists (Fields, 1982). Another is the "terminal thinking" noted earlier, in which youngsters come to believe that violent death is an inevitable fact of their lives, and respond accordingly, with fatalistic violence, depression, and antisocial behavior. Most terrorists, and many of our country's most violent criminals, have grown up in situations of chronic violence in which their behavior reflects the feelings of rage that often come from the experience of victimization, particularly among boys.

Families can do much to provide the emotional context for the necessary "processing" to make positive moral sense of danger, but it takes help from outside the home. If schoolteachers and other adult representatives of the community are unwilling or unable to demonstrate and teach higher order moral reasoning, or are intimidated if they try to do so, then the process of moral truncation that is "natural" to situations of violent conflict will proceed unimpeded.

In Northern Ireland, for example, both Protestant and Catholic teachers learned that if they tried to engage their students in dialogue that could promote higher order moral reasoning they would be silenced by extremist elements (Conroy, 1987). American urban gangs can have the same chilling effect if their threats come to dominate the institutions of a community. The prosocial forces in a community must remain in control of the schools, churches, neighborhood clubs, etc.

Children will continue to cope with difficult environments and maintain reservoirs of resilience so long as parents are not pushed beyond their capacity to absorb and deflect stress from children.

Once that point is exceeded, however, the development of young children deteriorates rapidly and markedly. Reservoirs of resilience become depleted. Day-to-day care breaks down, and rates of exploitation and victimization increase. Then moral development itself may be compromised.

The emerging problem of chronic gang violence poses a threat to youngsters that parallels other situations in which there is a dramatic and overwhelming destruction of the foundations of daily life. Erikson's (1976) study of an Appalachian community devastated by flood, speaks to what happens when a community loses faith with itself, when parents, teachers, and other adults are demoralized and powerless. "The major problem, for adults and children alike, is that the fears haunting them are prompted, not only by the memory of past terrors, but by a wholly realistic assessment of present dangers" (Erikson, 1976, p. 215).

What must we do? Part and parcel of any effort to make the streets and homes of children and youth safer is the willingness and ability of all adults to take charge of themselves. Evidence from World War II and from the Middle East indicates that the level of emotional upset displayed by adults in a child's life, *not the war situation per se,* was most important in predicting the child's response (Papanek, 1972). Parents who remained calm and in charge, confident and positive, were able to shield their children from much emotional harm. Teachers and other adults can play the same role.

CONCLUSION

Traumatized children need help to recover from their experiences (Terr, 1990). Emotionally disabled or immobilized adults are unlikely to offer children what they need. Such adults are inclined to engage in denial, to be emotionally inaccessible, and are prone to misinterpret the child's signals. Messages of safety are particularly important in establishing adults as sources of protection and authority for children living in conditions of threat and violence.

In Vygotsky's approach (1986), child development is fundamentally *social:* cognitive development proceeds at its best through the process of interactive teaching. He focuses on the Zone of Proximal Development: the difference between what the child can accomplish alone versus what the child can accomplish with the guidance of the teacher. How is this relevant to the child's ability to cope with trauma?

In the case of acute trauma (a single horrible incident that violates the normal reality of the child's world) the child needs help in believing that "things are back to normal." This is a relatively easy teaching task, this therapy of reassurance. But the child who lives with chronic trauma (e.g., the problem of community violence) needs something more. This child needs to be taught how to redefine the world in moral and structural terms.

The child needs assistance in "processing" the existing world if that child is to avoid drawing social and/or psychologically pathogenic conclusions: "the world is a hostile and dangerous place"; "adults have lost control of the world"; "kill or be killed"; "don't trust anyone"; "my enemies are less than human." Here the role of the adult as teacher is crucial for the well-being of the child, and for well-being of the community in which that child is to be a citizen.

The goal is to devise ways to help adults help youngsters wrestle with the powerful emotions that arise from living with chronic violence and to find alternative strategies for feeling safe and powerful (Garbarino et al., 1992). These methods include drawing, story-telling, dramatic play, and demonstrating openness to feelings, as strategies for helping children to "process" their experiences and feelings in a positive way (Garbarino and Manley, 1996).

On the one hand we have the commonsense assumption that children exposed to danger are destined for developmental difficulties: war is not good for children and other living things. On the other hand, we have the fact that children survive such danger and may even overcome its challenges in ways that enhance development. For this reason we must do something now for the children who are growing up amidst chronic violence. That something must include efforts to help them see positive paths ahead of them, paths that lead somewhere other than the next shoot-out (Garbarino, 1999).

REFERENCES

American Psychiatric Association (1994), *Diagnostic and Statistical Manual of Mental Disorders,* 4th ed. (DSM-IV). Washington, DC: American Psychiatric Press.
American Psychological Association (1993), *Summary Report of the American Psychological Association Committee on Violence and Youth.* Vol. 1. Washington, DC: American Psychological Association.
Bell, C. (1991), Traumatic stress and children in danger. *Health Care for the Poor and Underserved,* 2:175–188.
Conroy, J. (1987), *Belfast Diary.* Boston: Beacon Press.
Danieli, Y. (1988), The treatment and prevention of long-term effects and intergenerational transmission of victimization: A lesson from Holocaust survivors and their children. In: *Trauma and Its Wake,* ed. C. Figley. New York: Brunner/Mazel.
Davidson, J., & Smith, R. (1990), Traumatic experiences in psychiatric outpatients. *J. Traum. Stress Studies,* 3:459–475.
Dubrow, N., & Garbarino, J. (1989), Living in the war zone: Mothers and young children in a public housing development. *Child Welfare,* 68:3–20.
Erikson, K. (1976), *Everything in Its Path: Destruction of Community in the Buffalo Creek Flood.* New York: Simon & Schuster.
Fields, R. (1982), Terrorized into terrorist: Sequelae of PTSD in young victims. Paper presented at the meeting of the Society for Traumatic Stress Studies, New York, June.
Garbarino, J. (1995), *Raising Children in a Socially Toxic Environment: Childhood in the 1990s.* San Francisco: Jossey-Bass.
——— (1999), *Lost Boys: Why Our Sons Turn Violent and How We Can Save Them.* New York: Free Press.
——— Associates (1992), *Children and Families in the Social Environment.* New York: Aldine-de Gruyter.
——— Dubrow, N., Kostelny, K., & Pardo, C. (1992), *Children in Danger: Coping with the Consequences.* San Francisco: Jossey-Bass.
——— Kostelny, K., & Dubrow, N. (1991), *No Place to Be a Child: Growing Up in a War Zone.* Lexington, MA: Lexington Books.
——— Manley, J. (1996), Free play and captured play. *Internat. Play,* 4:123–132.

Groves, B., Zuckerman, B., Marans, S., & Cohen, D. (1993), Silent victims: Children who witness violence. *J. Amer. Med. Assn.*, 269:262–264.

Harris & Associates (1994), *Metropolitan Life Survey of the American Teacher: Violence in America's Public Schools.* Part II. New York: Metropolitan Life Insurance.

Herman, J. (1992), *Trauma and Recovery.* New York: Basic Books.

Kinzie, J., Sack, W., Angell, R., Manson, S., & Rath, B. (1986), The psychiatric effects of massive trauma on Cambodian children. *J. Amer. Acad. Child Psychiatry*, 25:370–376.

Kotlowitz, A. (1991), *There Are No Children Here.* New York: Doubleday.

Marans, S., & Cohen, D. (1993), Children and inner-city violence: Strategies for intervention. In: *Psychological Effects of War and Violence on Children*, ed. L. Leavitt & N. Fox. Hillsdale, NJ: Erlbaum, pp. 281–302.

Marin, C. (1989), Grief's children. WMAQ TV Documentary, Chicago, June 21.

Newsweek (1992), Growing up fast and frightened. March 9, p. 29.

Osofsky, J. (1995), The effects of exposure to violence on young children. *Amer. Psychologist*, 50:782–788.

Papanek, V. (1972), *Design for the Real World: Human Ecology and Social Change.* New York: Pantheon Books.

Price, J., & Desmond, S. (1987), The missing children issue: A preliminary examination of fifth-grade students' perceptions. *Amer. J. Diseases of Children*, 141:811–815.

Richters, J., & Martinez, P. (1993), The NIMH community violence project: Vol. 1. Children as victims of and as witnesses to violence. *Psychiatry*, 56:7–21.

Sameroff, A., Seifer, R., Barocas, R., Zax, M., & Greenspan, S. (1987), Intelligence quotient scores of 4-year-old children: Socio-environmental risk factors. *Pediatrics*, 79:343–350.

Terr, L. (1990), *Too Scared to Cry.* New York: Harper & Row.

Vygotsky, L. (1986), *Thought and Language.* Cambridge, MA: Massachusetts Institute of Technology Press.

10

Severe Physical Trauma in Adolescence

MAX SUGAR, M.D.

This chapter considers the emotional reactions of adolescents to physical trauma which is perceived as life-threatening.

DEFINITION

For adults, the term *railway compensation* neurosis was coined in the late nineteenth century, and *shell shock* was the term for emotional casualties of combat in World War I. The DSM-I (APA, 1952), and DSM-II (APA, 1968) listed traumatic neurosis, combat fatigue, and combat neurosis, but there was no listing for children or those adolescents younger than 18. Posttraumatic stress disorder relating to adults first appeared in the DSM-III (APA, 1980). It was not until DSM-III-R (APA, 1987) that diagnoses for children and all adolescents were included. Some changes in the criteria were made in DSM-IV (APA, 1994), but the major points, except for a broadening of trauma to include the perception of being life-threatening, remain essentially unchanged.

Erikson (1991) addresses the important question of blurred definitions whereby trauma is diagnosed simultaneously in PTSD

183

as a stimulus, the process, and the disordered state. He argues for more precision and limiting the term *trauma* to the emotional state resulting from the event. This would require two additional terms, one to specify the event, and another to designate the process.

INCIDENCE

From their surveys Bell and Jenkins (1991) calculated that about one-quarter to one-third of black youngsters under 18 in inner city Chicago had witnessed a shooting or a stabbing. Among middle and high school students, 35 percent had witnessed a stabbing, 39 percent had witnessed a shooting, and 24 percent had witnessed a killing. In Chicago in 1989, 20 percent of all homicide victims were aged between 11 and 20 years. The majority of victims were murdered by family members or friends (Bell and Jenkins, 1991).

Shaw and Harris (1994) noted that during the civil war in Mozambique, children and young adolescents who were coerced into becoming rebel soldiers had a very high percentage of PTSD. The authors helped to institute a reintegration program to draw the youngsters back into the mainstream of society and resume adolescent development.

Cosentino, Meyer-Bahlburg, Alpert, Weinberg, and Gaines (1995) estimate that one-quarter of all girls in the United States have been sexually abused before age 18, and one in ten boys have been similarly traumatized. In Canada, an estimated one in two females, and one in three males, have been victims of unwanted sexual acts during their lifetime; about 80 percent of these first occurred during childhood or youth; and in over 40 percent of all sexual homicides the victim was age 15 or younger (Minister of Supply and Services Canada, 1984, pp. 175–279).

Giaconia, Reinherz, Silverman, Pakiz, Frost, and Cohen (1995) found that among male and female high school seniors in a nonurban setting, more than two-fifths had experienced trauma; and that 6.3 percent had a lifetime diagnosis of PTSD, i.e., 14.5 percent of those with a qualifying trauma had a lifetime diagnosis of PTSD. Fifty percent of rape victims experienced PTSD. Twenty-seven percent of the seniors had been traumatized by age 14, and 12 percent had been traumatized by age 12. The median age of PTSD onset was 16 years, but in one-third the onset was by age 14. For 40 percent of the group, the duration of PTSD was one to three years. There was no difference found in the rate of PTSD related to socioeconomic status (SES).

Horowitz, Weine, and Jekel (1995) found a 67 percent rate of PTSD in urban female adolescents. Ten percent had been shot at; 21 percent had stabbed someone; 11 percent had been stabbed; 60 percent had assaulted someone; 28 percent had been assaulted; 9 percent were victims of unwanted sexual contact not in the home; 29 percent had been perpetrators of sexual contact in the home; 30 percent had been victims of unwanted sexual contact in the home; 37 percent had committed violent acts against family members before age 13; and 34 percent had themselves been victims of violence in the home before age 13.

REACTIONS TO ENVIRONMENTAL DISASTERS: FAMILY CONSIDERATIONS

A family fight and hostility between spouses often ensued postdisaster, even when there was no damage to the home or injury to its occupants (Crawshaw, 1963). Two years after the Buffalo Creek disaster the increase in teenage out-of-wedlock pregnancies correlated with the mothers' overall symptom severity and alcohol abuse. Increased delinquency was related to alcohol abuse by parents and alcohol-related imprisonment of parents, and depression in fathers. Fathers' rating for severity of depression correlated with that of adolescent sons, and their rating for anxiety correlated with the anxiety rating in sons and daughters, while belligerence in fathers correlated with depression in sons (Gleser,

Green, and Winget, 1981). Youngsters were more impaired if there was violence in the family atmosphere after the Buffalo Creek flood, and the distress of family members "tended to feed and grow on that of the other members" (Glesser et al., 1981; see chapter 11 of this volume for further aspects of the long-term effects).

Adolescents may appear to be comparatively self-sufficient and less vulnerable to further trauma postdisaster due to being physically more capable than either the aged or younger children. Adults experience a confused state with shock, disruption of their daily lives, threats to their integrity (physically, socially, and emotionally), after a trauma. Parents, rescue workers, or physicians often have their own posttraumatic difficulties (or use denial), which may interfere with observing or managing their adolescent's problems (Handford, Mayes, Mattison, Humphrey, Bagnato, Bixler, and Kales, 1986; Sugar, 1988a; Wraith, 1988; Yule and Udwin, 1991).

FACTORS CONTRIBUTING TO DISASTER EFFECTS

Bereavement or grief reactions in the survivors of disasters result from the death of relatives, friends, or pets. Physical pain or handicap follow injuries. Multiple, or secondary, traumatic events occur during and after a disaster and have a cumulative effect (Sugar, 1988b). These may include intrusions (such as by the media, lawyers, insurance agents, etc.), loss of job, home, and community, which can lead to an upheaval of family life which causes disruption in youngsters' development (Erikson, 1976; Sugar, 1988b, 1989; Wraith, 1988). With loss of community, home, friends, or possessions there is emotional disturbance, displacement from the home, and geographic relocation. All of these issues contribute to the teenager's emotional response and may interfere with development. These are listed in Table 10.1. Although focused on disaster, these may apply in various combinations to other physical trauma.

TABLE 10.1
Factors Contributing to Disaster Effects

Death
    Bereavement, Grief
Injuries
    Physical Pain, Threat of Disability
Threats of Further Trauma
    Fire
    Explosions
    Quakes
    Flooding
Multiple Secondary Trauma
    Intrusions
    Media, Legal
    Home Inspections
    Insurance Adjusters, Settlements
Associated Trauma and Loss
    Job
    Home
    Community
    Geographic Location
    Upheaval in Teen's Life
Interference with Development

ADOLESCENTS' RESPONSES TO DISASTER

There may be immediate nonspecific posttrauma effects. Among these are marked anxiety, brief crying or screaming, confusion with a shocklike state, disorganization, frozen or inhibited movement, apathy, a sense of hopelessness, withdrawal, disturbed appetite, insomnia, separation anxiety, and school refusal.

The nonspecific reactions that may be evident in a few days or weeks after a trauma (Terr, 1979, 1983; Gleser et al., 1981; Sugar, 1989) are listed in Tables 10.2 and 10.3. These would fit the diagnosis of acute stress reaction or PTSD.

Following a physical trauma there is a high risk that adolescents may engage in vandalism, malicious mischief, disorderly conduct, and assault (Adams and Adams, 1984); brawling, robbery, delinquency, increased use and abuse of alcohol, drugs, and tobacco

TABLE 10.2

Adolescents' Response to Disaster Trauma

Immediate Nonspecific Symptoms
Marked Anxiety
Screaming, Shouting, Crying
Confusion
Shocklike State
Disorganization
Frozen or Inhibited Affect
Apathy
Sense of Hopelessness
Withdrawal
Disturbed Appetite
Insomnia
Separation Anxiety
School Refusal

TABLE 10.3

Adolescents' Response to Disaster Trauma

Nonspecific Symptoms a Few Weeks after Trauma	
Insomnia	Psychosomatic Symptoms
Nightmares	Hostility
Somnambulism	Irritability
Clinging	Anxiety
Lack of Personal Responsibility	Violent Behavior
	Brooding
Decreased School Performance	Omens with Negative Predictions
Withdrawal	Decreased Goals
Apathy	Foreshortening of Future
Loss of Interest	Pessimism
Attention and Concentration Problems	Guilt about Survival
	Hypertension

(Erikson, 1976; Gleser et al., 1981). Early dissociative reactions (i.e., sudden, temporary altered states of consciousness, identity, or motor behavior) may occur, and years later there may be multiple personality organization.

Adolescents may have symptoms specific to the trauma such as fears, depression, anxiety, and belligerence (Green, Korol, Grace, Vary, Leonard, Gleser, and Smitson-Cohen, 1992), recall of, and reexperiencing with various stimuli, phobias about these with startle (diffuse motor) responses, risky behavior, distortions and misperceptions in time with sequencing, duration, and time skew. Intrusive symptoms and amnesia were noted in some adolescents by Yule and Williams (1989) and me, which is contrary to the findings by Garmezy and Rutter (1985). Yule and Williams (1989) and I have observed flashbacks and avoidance in adolescents with PTSD.

Since adolescents' cognitive ability is greater than that of children they can assess and perceive trauma more readily. Their responses are based on their own perceptions of the trauma which are governed by their cognitive, emotional and physical developmental level, but they may also be influenced by family factors (Frederick, 1985; Handford et al., 1986; Gleser et al., 1991; Honig, Grace, Lindy, Newman, and Titchener, 1993). Those who are geographically closer to the site of the disaster have a more extreme or severe reaction with decreased ability to concentrate and may have memory interferences. This also applies to the injured; those with injured, dead, or missing relatives or friends; those with poor or disorganized living conditions; those relocated geographically or separated from their family; and those intruded on by strangers.

GENDER DIFFERENCES

Adolescent girls show more distress than boys following a disaster (Dohrenwend, Dohrenwend, Warheit, Bartlett, Goldstein, Goldstein, and Martin, 1981; Gleser et al., 1981; Ollendick and Hoffman, 1983; Milgram, Toubiana, Klingman, Raviv, and Goldstein, 1988; Zeidner, 1993). Giaconia et al. (1995) found that males and females were equally likely to experience the effects of trauma; however, females were six times more likely to develop subsequent PTSD. They felt, however, that this was consistent with the male pattern of reporting every type of PTSD symptom less frequently than females.

Even if hostile and antisocial behavior have not been part of their previous pattern, male adolescents tend to discharge angry and anxious feelings in that fashion posttrauma. Compared to females they use significantly more denial and experience more difficulty in engaging, and remaining, in therapy. Decreased motivation for therapy in teenage females may also be due to feeling threatened by revealing their symptoms since these reflect a sense of loss of control (similar to feelings about menses).

DIAGNOSES

While resilient youngsters may show no evidence of emotional distress from trauma, some may have responses which they deny and suppress. There are others who have frequent frightening dreams of the trauma, dissociative episodes, intrusive thoughts, amnesia, hypervigilance, hyperarousal, fugues, or later on develop multiple personality. The connection between the trauma and the adolescents' poor academic performance, misconduct, increased rate of unwed pregnancies, delinquency, vandalism, alcoholism, rowdiness, and substance abuse may be overlooked.

In some posttrauma youngsters there may be insufficient findings for a diagnosis despite the fact that they have some symptoms. An acute stress reaction may last for a short time. But for some, a generalized anxiety disorder, a major depression, an adjustment disorder, conduct disorder, PTSD, or other diagnoses may follow.

Posttraumatic Stress Disorder may be seen immediately posttrauma in some adolescents and last several months or for years after, but the connection between their symptoms and the trauma may go unnoticed for many years. Prior individual or family psychopathology compounds the problem (Handford et al., 1986). However, as DSM-IV indicates, a prior history of psychopathology is not required for a diagnosis of PTSD, and as section A indicates, this may happen to anyone (American Psychiatric Association, 1994).

CASE EXAMPLE 1

A 15-year-old girl, whose neck and back were injured in an oil refinery explosion that blew her home apart, had thought intrusion, flashbacks, recurrent thoughts, repetitious dreams, and nightmares about the disaster. She developed increased appetite and weight. She became irritable and restless, fussed with her siblings, and kept distant from peers. She had great sensitivity to noise and avoided it (e.g., movies), as well as stimuli that reminded her of the disaster. She showed denial, but was aware of her sadness. After the disaster she felt peers and teachers picked on her. She pursued repetitive, meaningless activities (e.g., repeatedly writing her name). Her diagnosis was PTSD. She was uncooperative and hostile about psychotherapy.

CASE EXAMPLE 2

This 13-year-old male injured his neck and jaw in a disaster and was still in a neck brace several months later. He was withdrawn, less talkative and friendly than before the accident and had insomnia. He had discipline problems caused by daydreaming about the disaster in class. His other symptoms fulfilled criteria for a diagnosis of PTSD, but he was opposed to therapy.

CASE EXAMPLE 3

A 13-year-old male was severely injured during an industrial explosion that destroyed his home. The family was evacuated safely and moved to another town to temporary, cramped quarters without a phone. For many months afterward, there were poor arrangements for daily needs, school, recreation, etc. He complained of back and neck aches. He had not resumed school several months later.

One night while mother was experiencing an anxiety attack, her mate insisted on sexual intercourse. When she refused and he persisted, she screamed for help and all five children came into the bedroom. When this boy attacked the father-surrogate with a knife, the father-surrogate took it from him. The mother feared the boy would be killed, but the boy escaped their quarters and ran for the police two-and-a-half blocks away. When the police appeared the man had fled with the only set of keys after locking the family inside. Later when he returned, after he had been drinking, they feared he would kill them. The mother was interested in the youngster's continued psychiatric treatment, but he rejected it.

This case illustrates some of the multiple trauma (dislocation, school, and community disruptions) after a disaster (Sugar, 1988b) as well as the inappropriate behavior of the father-figure (drinking, violence, denial of his mate's distress), and the disrupted family of an early adolescent with violent behavior, PTSD, and a conduct disorder.

CASE EXAMPLE 4

A late teenager survived a nighttime auto accident in which his girl friend and the other driver, who caused the accident, were killed. He had some injuries to his limbs for which he received excellent orthopedic treatment, but no psychiatric assessment was done. About two years after the event he was persuaded to seek psychiatric treatment.

Although he was intoxicated during the accident, he saw and recalled gruesome details of her demise. He had flashbacks, thought intrusion, and some amnesia. His schoolwork was poor, he was mistrustful, aggressive, unsettled as to vocational goals and friendships, irritable, had loss of appetite, insomnia (early and midsleep), anxiety attacks, fears of dying while driving at night, nightmares, feelings of guilt, numbness, disinterest, and a sense of a foreshortened future. He noted a change from having agreeable and compliant responses to his parents to a state of constant verbal clashes or silence with them. Risky behavior had increased.

Prior to the accident he had severely abused alcohol, and been involved in three car wrecks in which he was the driver. Continued alcohol abuse led to a brief exposure to Alcoholics Anonymous without any habit change. He was diagnosed as PTSD with alcohol abuse.

These cases illustrate some of the range of reactions, symptoms, and diagnoses in adolescent victims of trauma.

SEQUELAE OF TRAUMA IN ADOLESCENCE

Erikson (1976) observed that two years after the Buffalo Creek disaster the teenagers had an increase in delinquency. Gleser et al. (1981) found that two years after that disaster, those aged 12 to 14 had more symptoms than younger children and fewer symptoms than adults, but the 16- to 20-year-olds had the most severe symptoms along with belligerence, depression, and anxiety. Before the flood, hypertension was present in 9 percent of black males, 2 percent of white males, 23 percent of black females, and 8 percent of white females. Two years postflood, 25 percent of white adolescent females and 41 percent of white adolescent males had hypertension. These rates for white adolescents indicate a marked increase, and a reversal of the usual black:white ratio.

Two years after the Buffalo Creek disaster, the youngsters were smoking, drinking, racing vehicles, robbing, and brawling in groups. Those 12 to 15 years old were more belligerent postflood (based on separation or death of parent) than other teens, and 75 percent of them had insomnia. There was a 12 percent increase in delinquency. Females had a 9 percent increase in teen pregnancy, and were more disturbed than males at every age. Black male and female adolescents were less disturbed than whites. Four years after the disaster some adolescents showed more impairment than they had shown in prior years, and more than 30 percent suffered debilitating symptoms (Gleser et al., 1981).

At the 20-year follow-up of youngsters who were 12 to 16 years old at the time of the Buffalo Creek disaster (Honig et al., 1993), some of the group were not functioning well, while most of them manifested adaptive character traits related to the disaster. The authors felt that the family's responses to the flood and its aftermath were closely tied to the evolution of the youngsters' adaptive patterns.

A residual level of anxiety was found in adolescents one-and-a-half years after the evacuation at Three Mile Island (Handford et al., 1986). In a life-threatening situation among Americans in a foreign country, Rigamer (1986) observed increased denial, suspicion, xenophobia, prejudice, and intellectualization in adolescents. Following a school bus disaster, Toubiana, Milgram, Strich, and Edelstein (1988) recorded withdrawal, school refusal, and separation anxiety symptoms in early adolescents. Yule and Williams (1991) noted that higher levels of disaster symptoms of 50 percent and 75 percent, were reported by youngsters age 11 to 15 after a shipwreck when they were seen separately from parents and teachers, respectively.

After a disaster 60 percent of those under age 18 had PTSD according to Frederick (1985). Children 11 to 14 had sleep and appetite disruption, rebelliousness, fighting, withdrawal, loss of interest, need for excess attention, physical and psychosomatic symptoms, and school misbehavior. Among the 14- to 18-year-olds there was also amenorrhea or dysmenorrhea in the females; both sexes experienced apathy, agitation, decreased interest in the opposite sex; and irresponsible or delinquent behavior.

Bell and Jenkins (1991) observed that mourning for the victim may be complicated by anxiety triggered by the memory of the event witnessed, and by rage and revenge toward the perpetrator. The witness has problems about identification with the aggressor, avoiding becoming a victim, and retaliating. They recommended a screening program for all youngsters in inner city schools.

Haviland, Sonne, and Woods (1995) observed that the severity of PTSD was greater in sexually abused males and females than those who had been physically abused. They found that object relations and reality testing disturbances were common. The degree of insecure attachment, egocentricity, and disturbances in reality testing were correlated with the severity of PTSD symptoms.

Giaconia et al. (1995) noted that by age 18 the seniors mentioned earlier who were exposed to trauma and had PTSD had much poorer functioning than the seniors who had trauma without PTSD. Those with that diagnosis had interpersonal, externalizing problems; increased suicidal thoughts and attempts; more sick days; and their general level of functioning was less compared to those who had not experienced trauma. The trauma-only group also had significant problems similar to the PTSD group with health, academics, suicidal ideation, and suicide attempts. For the adolescents with PTSD there was an increased risk of having major depression, and two-fifths of those with PTSD had that diagnosis within a year of PTSD onset.

There was also a much higher risk of substance dependence in those with PTSD, since 67 percent of them were on drugs within one year after its onset, and 46 percent had alcohol dependency within one year after the onset of PTSD. For those with trauma-only, there was an increased risk of alcohol dependence and drug dependence. The results from this study are not applicable to the population of youth at large since the subjects were all white from a working- or middle-class socioeconomic background (Giaconia et al., 1995).

If there was violence in the home and the community, a community trauma was compounded. There was a sense of collective traumatization from hearing about traumatic events (rape, mugging shootings, deaths, stabbings, serious accidents, friends and enemies being killed, relatives being killed, boyfriends being killed). Adolescents mistrusted their own family members. Their interpersonal relationships and identity formation were altered. Their future orientation was decreased as was their hope that life would improve (Horowitz et al., 1995).

Van der Kolk (1997) states that there is evidence that there may be amnesia for some, or all, aspects of trauma, as well as flashback memory for particular episodes. The latter does not necessarily bestow accuracy on the scene of trauma.

Acute and chronic emotional illness with lengthy impairment may be the legacy of psychic trauma, and these require an extended period of treatment. The children of Chowchilla with their continuing trauma effects four to five years afterward (Terr, 1983), the findings at the twenty-year follow-up on Buffalo Creek by Honig et al. (1993; and see chapter 11), and the views of Koenig (1964) and Sugar (chapter 14) about adolescent survivors of the Holocaust, support this notion.

APPROACHES TO ADOLESCENT DISASTER VICTIMS

Mild transient feelings of depersonalization and derealization appear to be particularly common in adolescence (Bernstein and Putnam, 1986). From experience with youngsters in a disaster it seems that perhaps the stress of a disaster and the reaction to it are experienced as depersonalization or derealization by adolescents. They may then disavow or deny their symptoms of distress, making them less available for psychotherapy. This may be augmented by a "macho" defense, and aided (without awareness) by parental or teacher denial. The correlation between their anger and wish for revenge (for losses and disruptions) seems evident in their symptomatic behavior but may be overlooked. The adolescent's denial may also be a feature which aids pursuit of retaliation.

Just as there is an auxiliary ego and a parental protective barrier provided to the infant by its mother in infancy, so, too, this protective barrier continues, but in lessening degrees, through childhood and adolescence. Regardless of the degree of independence achieved, most adolescents still look to this support, guidance, and protection from parents in times of stress or trauma. However, when trauma of such a degree occurs that it leads to an acute stress reaction or PTSD, the adolescent feels abandoned by, and loses trust in, the parents. With faith in parents' and their own invincibility decreased or nullified by trauma, especially in a disaster, there is often a sense of distrust, and hopelessness with apathy, that makes it difficult for adolescents to trust another adult, accept, or appear for, psychiatric evaluation, or engage in therapy.

Adolescents should be given more information than younger children, along with an appeal to their cognitive abilities and experiences, while respecting their defenses (Rigamer, 1986). Tenth graders who spoke about their feelings before an anticipated earthquake (which did not occur) had increased symptoms before the anticipated date, but they had a significant decrease in symptoms of stress at the second interview at a later date. If the youngsters' families had prepared them for the earthquake, the adolescents had more stress symptoms before the anticipated date of the earthquake and a much larger decrease in symptoms afterward compared to those whose families did not prepare them (Kiser, Heston, Hickerson, Millsap, Nunn, and Pruitt, 1993). Screening scales are of limited value without detailed individual interviews (Yule and Udwin, 1991).

All trauma victims should have brief group therapy and crisis management immediately after the event. In some areas the states or local disaster agencies usually provide this for six to twelve weeks on a weekly or biweekly basis (Sugar, 1989). Toubiana et

al. (1988) felt that crisis management was useful and that some
adolescents responded to such efforts.

If the youngster's symptoms continue unabated, despite reassurance, support, and medication for several weeks after the disaster, then psychiatric consultation is imperative. When risky or
dangerous behavior occurs following a trauma, immediate psychiatric attention is needed.

Group therapy with adolescents postdisaster is helpful, but the
majority of youngsters still had "significant psychological morbidity" after more than a year of treatment in a group (Yule and
Williams, 1989). Individual, group, and family therapy (Gleser et
al., 1981) should be used as needed along with medication. A
parallel parents' therapy group may be helpful.

Since anger usually accompanies loss (Bowlby, 1958) and it is
apparent posttrauma, it becomes an issue early in therapy and a
resistance. There may also be an admixture in the youngster's
symptoms of projection and identification with the aggressor
when the disaster is man-made.

CONCLUSION

This presentation reviews the cognitive, emotional, physical, and
behavioral effects on adolescents involved in trauma which causes
posttraumatic stress disorder. Group delinquent behavior, increased substance abuse, academic decline, unwed adolescent
pregnancy, increased vandalism, violence, and risk-taking may en-
sue along with raised blood pressure. Case illustrations provide
some highlights of such consequences. The long-term effects include problems in academics, vocation, interpersonal relations,
substance abuse, continued PTSD symptoms, and major depression.

Recognition of adolescents' posttrauma denial and symptoms
is a major determinant for them to have an evaluation and treatment. Their parents and other caregivers may have problems in

recognizing or supporting their need for therapy. It seems that with the present state of affairs in urban war zones and the high risk for trauma, even in nonurban settings, exposure to trauma should be considered as a possibility already present when assessing adolescents with various symptoms that seem to be related to trauma. Screening for trauma victims in violent areas of inner cities may be a positive preventive and therapeutic measure.

Adolescents who are physically traumatized, whether with PTSD or with posttrauma anxiety, are not motivated for treatment, which adds to their difficulties in obtaining help. There may be considerable countertransference problems in treating these youngsters. Further observations of long-term developmental effects and treatment outcome are needed.

REFERENCES

Adams, P. R., & Adams, G. R. (1984), Mount Saint Helens's ashfall: Evidence for a disaster stress reaction. *Amer. Psychologist*, 39:252–260.

American Psychiatric Association (1952), *Diagnostic and Statistical Manual of Mental Disorders* (DSM-I). Washington, DC: American Psychiatric Association.

——— (1968), *Diagnostic and Statistical Manual of Mental Disorders*, 2nd ed. (DSM-II). Washington, DC: American Psychiatric Association.

——— (1980), *Diagnostic and Statistical Manual of Mental Disorders*, 3rd ed. (DSM-III). Washington, DC: American Psychiatric Press.

——— (1987), *Diagnostic and Statistical Manual of Mental Disorders*, 3rd ed. rev. (DSM-III-R). Washington, DC: American Psychiatric Press.

——— (1994), *Diagnostic and Statistical Manual of Mental Disorders*, 4th ed. (DSM-IV). Washington, DC: American Psychiatric Press.

Bell, C. C., & Jenkins, E. J. (1991), Traumatic stress and children. *J. Health Care for the Poor Underserved*, 2:175–185.

Bernstein, E. M., & Putnam, F. W. (1986), Development, reliability and validity of a Dissociation Scale. *J. Nerv. & Ment. Dis.*, 174:727–735.

Bowlby, J. (1958), The nature of the child's tie to his mother. *Internat. J. Psycho-Anal.*, 39:1–23.

Cosentino, C. E., Meyer-Bahlburg, H. F. L., Alpert, J. L., & Weinberg, S. L., & Gaines, R. (1995), Sexual behavior problems and psychopathology symptoms in sexually abused girls. *J. Amer. Acad. Child Adol. Psychiatry*, 34:1033–1043.

Crawshaw, R. (1963), Reaction to disaster. *Arch. Gen. Psychiatry*, 9:157–162.

Dohrenwend, B. P., Dohrenwend, B. S., Warheit, G. J., Bartlett, G. S., Goldstein, R. L., Goldstein, K., & Martin, J. L. (1981), Stress in the community: A report to the President's Commission on the accident at Three Mile Island. *Ann. NY Acad. Sci.*, 365:159–174.

Erikson, K. (1976), *Everything in Its Path*. New York: Simon & Schuster.

—— (1991), Notes on trauma and community. *Amer. Imago*, 48:455–472.

Frederick, C. J. (1985), Children traumatized by catastrophic situations. In: *Post-Traumatic Stress Disorder in Children*, ed. S. Eth & R. S. Pynoos. Washington, DC: American Psychiatric Press.

Garmezy, N., & Rutter, M. (1985), Acute reactions to stress. In: *Child Psychiatry: Modern Approaches*, 2nd ed., ed. M. Rutter & L. Hersov. Oxford: Blackwell.

Giaconia, R. M., Reinherz, H. Z., Silverman, A. B., Pakiz, B., Frost, A. K., & Cohen, E. (1995), Traumas and posttraumatic stress disorder in a community population of older adolescents. *J. Amer. Acad. Child & Adol. Psychiatry*, 34:1369–1380.

Gleser, G. C., Green, B. L., & Winget, C. (1981), *Prolonged Psychosocial Effects of Disaster: A Study of Buffalo Creek*. New York: Academic Press.

Green, B. L., Korol, M., Grace, M. C., Vary, M. G., Leonard, A. C., Gleser, G. C., & Smitson-Cohen, S. (1992), Children and disaster: Age, gender and parental effects on PTSD symptoms. *J. Amer. Acad. Child & Adol. Psychiatry*, 30:945–951.

Handford, H. A., Mayes, S. D., Mattison, R. E., Humphrey, F. J., Bagnato, S., Bixler, E. O., & Kales, J. D. (1986), Child and parent reaction to the Three Mile Island nuclear accident. *J. Amer. Acad. Child Psychiatry*, 25:346–356.

Haviland, M. G., Sonne, J. L., & Woods, L. (1995), Beyond posttraumatic stress disorder: Object relations and reality testing disturbances in physically and sexually abused adolescents. *J. Amer. Acad. Child & Adol. Psychiat.*, 34:1054–1060.

Honig, R. E., Grace, M. C., Lindy, J. D., Newman, C. J., & Titchener, J. L. (1993), Portraits of survival. A twenty year follow-up of the children of Buffalo Creek. *The Psychoanalytic Study of the Child*, 48:327–355. New Haven, CT: Yale University Press.

Horowitz, K., Weine, S., & Jekel, J. (1995), PTSD symptoms in urban adolescent girls: Compounded community trauma. *J. Amer. Acad. Child & Adol. Psychiatry*, 34:1353–1361.

Kiser, L., Heston, J., Hickerson, S., Millsap, P., Nunn, W., & Pruitt, D. (1993), Anticipatory stress in children and adolescents. *Amer. J. Psychiatry*, 150:87–92.

Koenig, W. K. (1964), Chronic or persistent identity diffusion. *Amer. J. Psychiatry*, 120:1081–1084.

Milgram, N. A., Toubiana, Y. H., Klingman, A., Raviv, A., & Goldstein, I. (1988), Situational exposure and personal loss in children's acute and chronic stress reactions to a school bus disaster. *J. Traum. Stress*, 1:330–352.

Minister of Supply and Services, Canada (1984), *Sexual Offenses Against Children*, Vol. 1. Ottawa: Canadian Government Publishing.

Ollendick, D. G., & Hoffman, M. (1983), Assessment of psychological reactions in disaster victims. *J. Commun. Psychology*, 10:157–167.

Rigamer, E. F. (1986), Psychological management of children in a national crisis. *J. Amer. Acad. Child Psychiatry*, 25:364–369.

Shaw, J. A., & Harris, J. J. (1994), Children of war and children at war: Child victims of terrorism in Mozambique. In: *Individual and Community Responses to Trauma and Disaster: The Structure of Human Chaos*, ed. R. J. Ursano, B. B. McCaughey, & C. S. Fullerton. Cambridge, UK: Cambridge University Press.

Sugar, M. (1988a), A preschooler in a disaster. *Amer. J. Psychother.*, 42:619–629.

—— (1988b), The multiple trauma in a disaster. In: *The Child in His Family. Perilous Development: Child Raising and Identity Formation Under Stress*, ed. E. J. Anthony & C. Chiland. York: John Wiley.

—— (1989), Children in a disaster—An overview. *Child Psychiatry Hum. Develop.*, 19:163–179.

Terr, L. C. (1979), Children of Chowchilla. *The Psychoanalytic Study of the Child*, 35:547–623. New Haven, CT: Yale University Press.

—— (1983), Chowchilla revisited: The effects of psychic trauma four years after a school-bus kidnapping. *Amer. J. Psychiatry*, 140:1543–1550.

Toubiana, Y. H., Milgram, N. A., Strich, Y., & Edelstein, A. (1988), Crisis intervention in a school community disaster: Principles and practices. *J. Commun. Psychology*, 16:228–240.

van der Kolk, B. A. (1997), Posttraumatic stress disorder and memory. *Psychiatric Times*, March:54–55.

Wraith, R. (1988), Experiences in children of workers in emergency services and disaster situations. Paper presented at the International Conference on Dealing with Stress and Trauma in Emergency Services, Melbourne, Australia.

Yule, W., & Udwin, O. (1991), Screening child survivors for post-traumatic stress disorders: Experiences from the "Jupiter" sinking. *Brit. J. Clin. Psychology*, 30:131–138.

—— Williams, R. M. (1989), Post-traumatic stress reactions in children. *J. Traum. Stress*, 3:279–295.

Zeidner, M. (1993), Coping with disaster: The case of Israeli adolescents under threat of missile attack. *J. Youth & Adol.*, 22:89–108.

11

Assessing the Long-Term Effects of Disasters Occurring during Childhood and Adolescence

Questions of Perspective and Methodology

RICHARD G. HONIG, M.D., MARY C. GRACE, M.ED., M.S., JACK D. LINDY, M.D., C. JANET NEWMAN, M.D., JAMES L. TITCHENER, M.D.

In an earlier paper describing the effects of the Buffalo Creek Flood, the current authors (1993) posed the question, "But could anyone ever know all that happened in that valley on that cold, wet, bleak Saturday (February 26, 1972)? We have a patchwork, a collage of reports of people who witnessed portions of the disaster from different perspectives" (p. 328). As researchers with a twenty-year history following the survivors of Buffalo Creek, we

The project was supported by the Research Fund of the Cincinnati Psychoanalytic Institute. The authors would like to thank Ms. Susan Bailey for her assistance with this project.

are now compelled to pose a similar question, this time regarding the possibility of knowing all the effects of this disaster. Ongoing Buffalo Creek research, which taken in its totality is perhaps the most thorough psychological investigation of a disaster ever undertaken, is itself now a collage that seems to demonstrate that our assessment of the effects of the flood, too, are a matter of perspective and the methodology to which a particular perspective gives rise. This has led to caution about what we think we know and a growing awareness of the possible limiting effects of the instruments and techniques used to assess the effects of trauma.

From its inception, the multidisciplinary team which followed the survivors of the Buffalo Creek disaster has included two branches: (1) a group of psychodynamically oriented clinicians, and (2) a group of empirically focused, group level researchers. Those questions which have driven the research throughout these many years have emanated from the productive dialogue that has evolved between these two groups.

This current study focuses on the long-term effects of the Buffalo Creek disaster on the child and adolescent survivors and the degree to which a standardized research methodology for group level assessment is sufficient to diagnose the presence of Post-Traumatic Stress Disorder (PTSD) and other trauma-related symptoms in a survivor population. This research focus was an outgrowth of the authors' previously reported twenty-year follow-up of the children of Buffalo Creek, "Portraits of Survival" (1993). That study itself was born of questions about perspective and methodology raised by our colleagues in the NIMH funded follow-up of the children of Buffalo Creek conducted by the University of Cincinnati Traumatic Stress Study Center (Green, 1987).

Utilizing a standardized methodology (structured clinical interview for DSM-III, SCID) to assess levels of psychopathology among ninety-nine child survivors at seventeen years postflood, Green, Grace, Vary, Kramer, Gleser, and Leonard (1994) found that both PTSD and other psychopathology had sharply declined from levels reported by Gleser, Green, and Winget (1978) at two years postflood. They tentatively concluded that these child and adolescent survivors appeared to have "recovered." However, they were not content to accept their group level findings as the final word on the long-term effects of the flood for any particular survivor. They conceived another study to explore, in a small number of individual survivors, the long-term meaning, which the flood may have taken on in their lives, as well as the flood's impact on adaptation and personality formation as further emotional development unfolded. Those researchers felt that the standardized methodology that had been used in the NIMH study would not be adequate to address the issues raised by this shift in perspective because of its focus on group level findings. They selected, therefore, a psychodynamically focused clinical interview as the most appropriate technique to explore questions of adaptation and development.

To carry out this more in-depth exploration of the lingering effects of the flood, a separate team of clinicians was formed that was expert in the conduct of the psychodynamic interview. Subjects were interviewed with a one- to two-hour open-ended format in which the flood and its sequelae through the life cycle were the sole focus. As interviews were conducted with a number of child and adolescent survivors, who had now become young adults, the authors discovered that the flood had enduring effects on these individuals despite the fact that they had not met criteria for PTSD in their prior interview using the Structured Clinical Interview for DSM-III-R (SCID). They concluded that the presence or absence of a residual posttraumatic stress disorder was not the only, or perhaps even the most important, measure of the long-term impact of a traumatic event occurring during the years of childhood and adolescence. They found such long-term effects often took the shape of persistent character traits which may have originated as coping responses to the trauma. These characterological patterns were seen as more or less adaptational and more or less defensive from the standpoint of subsequent emotional development and the individuals' capacity to confront later stressful events (Honig et al., 1993).

Although the psychodynamic interviewing techniques utilized for this study were chosen for their sensitivity to just such issues of meaning and adaptation, the research team was intrigued by another, incidental finding which ultimately gave rise to the study now being reported. In certain of the subjects, active PTSD symptomatology was elicited that had not been picked up by means of the SCID interview utilized in the seventeen-year follow-up study. A decision was made to investigate this finding further with a more thorough review of the research videotapes, now with a particular eye to the discovery of persistent PTSD symptomatology. As more evidence emerged that PTSD symptoms had not been reported by survivors in response to the structured SCID interview, the question arose as to which type of symptoms seemed sensitive to discovery by means of the psychodynamic interview, and what about this methodology, as contrasted with the SCID interview, allowed these additional PTSD symptoms to emerge.

Returning to the psychodynamic clinical interview in this investigation has brought the Buffalo Creek research full circle, in that the psychodynamic clinical interview was the technique used to generate the enormous body of information from which the original Buffalo Creek studies emerged. By way of further introduction to this present study, a description of the flood itself and a brief summary of the methodology and findings of prior Buffalo Creek studies is in order.

THE FLOOD

Buffalo Creek is a small mining community located in an eighteen-mile-long valley in Logan County, West Virginia. In late February 1972, it had been raining for several days and there was concern about the safety of the slag dam crudely created through the dumping of refuse at the top of the valley. A coal mine delivered to its tipple 90 percent waste and 10 percent coal. For years, rumors had abounded that the dam might give way and "God only knew what would happen then." However, the coal company, the major employer in the valley, assured the residents there was nothing to fear.

Early on Saturday morning, February 26th, the dam did collapse, pouring millions of gallons of water and sludge into the valley below and creating a speeding wall of black mud estimated to have been thirty to forty feet high over the creek bed. The water/mud literally caromed its way between the steep valley walls carrying along in its path houses, trailers, autos, and human bodies, leaving 125 people dead, 4,000 homeless, and the landscape and community devastated. After many weeks, the worst of the debris was still being cleared away.

The trauma was compounded by ill-conceived relocation efforts that included the separation of kin and nuclear families, multiple moves of families, and the decision of the West Virginia government to build a new highway up the middle of the valley, preventing many people from returning to their land. The situation did not really stabilize for several years. During this period, residents who felt that the fault for this disaster lay with the coal company for constructing the dam in an unsafe manner joined in a lawsuit that included claims of "psychic impairment" as well as property damage and wrongful death. Under the direction of Dr. James Titchener, the University of Cincinnati Department of Psychiatry became involved in a lawsuit for the plaintiffs and conducted extensive individual psychiatric interviews and family assessments with 381 adult and 207 child survivors between eighteen and twenty-six months after the flood (Green, Lindy, Grace, Gleser, Leonard, Korol, and Winget, 1990; Honig et al., 1993).

The lawsuit was eventually settled out of court for $13.5 million, which included an unprecedented $8 million for psychic impairment (Stern, 1976). This settlement represented a landmark recognition that survivors, who may not have been physically injured, were in every sense victims. The scope of the psychiatric evaluations carried out for this lawsuit was also unprecedented in disaster research and became a legacy to a generation of Buffalo Creek researchers. Just as the lawsuit set a legal precedent, the initial

Buffalo Creek research effort that commenced shortly after the settlement, and focused both on the adult and child survivor populations, broke new ground in the understanding of the psychological consequences of disaster.

HISTORY OF THE BUFFALO CREEK RESEARCH

Approximately two years after the flood, teams were assembled to conduct the psychiatric evaluations for the survivors' lawsuit. These teams consisted of general and child psychiatrists, psychologists and social workers, all University of Cincinnati (UC) Department of Psychiatry clinicians who shared a psychoanalytic orientation. The teams visited their assigned families in the valley itself and conducted their interviews in the survivors' mobile homes and those houses that were left standing (Titchener and Kapp, 1976).

The conduct of the interviews was described as follows:

We began each evaluation with a family interview in which we asked the survivors to talk about experiences on the "day of the black water" and during the weeks and months that followed. As they talked, we were able to see beyond the immediate clinical phenomenon to these people's underlying feelings and their ways of coping with them. The family sessions were followed by psychoanalytically oriented individual interviews with each family member, conducted in back yards, living rooms, or on porches [p. 296].

For the adult subjects, the individual assessments which followed the family interview utilized a semistructured format to elicit the symptoms and emotions both immediately following the disaster and at the time of the interview. Also noted were changes in work motivation, interpersonal relations outside and inside the family, current dreams and reactions to rain storms. Where children were to be evaluated, an outline of each child's developmental history before and after the flood was obtained from the mother and passed on to the child psychiatrist. Whenever possible, children were seen in their own rooms where they were encouraged to recall their own experience of the flood, which had often been submerged or inhibited in the earlier part of the interview amidst the outpourings of the adult family members. Discussion included descriptions of past and present family life, school experiences, and future hopes. In addition, fantasy eliciting techniques, including storytelling and drawing, were utilized. Special educators obtained school data to correct or confirm parental impressions of changes in academic performance postdisaster (Newman, 1976).

As the lawsuit was being settled, this unprecedented record of postdisaster adjustment began to be mined for its enormous research potential. Separate teams studied the clinical records of both the adult and child survivor populations.

Results of the initial adult study (Titchener and Kapp, 1976) found traumatic neurotic symptoms to be present in 80 percent of the survivors and concluded as well that there need not be any preexisting psychiatric impairment in order for the postdisaster syndrome to become disabling and chronic. This postdisaster symptom complex included intrusive memories and dreams of the flood, heightened vigilance and phobic experience at times of flood reminders, as well as depression and rage.

In addition to this symptom picture, the original adult study found posttraumatic character changes to be equally widespread. Those character changes were collectively described as psychic numbing and included chronic depressive features and survivor guilt, both contributing to lives dominated by self-denial, shrinking energies, dampened socialization, lack of hope, and a dissolution of self-confidence. These character changes were seen as protecting the victims from reexperiencing the traumatic state and the accompanying affects of fear, rage, and helplessness, while at the same time preserving symptom patterns, forcing changes in life-style, and interfering with effective recovery, which would have required active recall and mastery of the painful memories.

As to the earliest Buffalo Creek child studies, Newman's (1976) findings indicated that most of the children were also significantly emotionally impaired two years after the flood. The most prominent features of the children's postdisaster syndrome included troubling and intrusive imagery, terrifying nightmares, increased nervous tension, withdrawal, depression, enuresis, hypochondriasis, and failing grades at school. The common heritage of these children appeared to be a "modified sense of reality, increased vulnerability to future stresses, an altered sense of the powers within the self, and a precocious awareness of fragmentation and death" (p. 312).

Even as these original Buffalo Creek adult and child studies were being published, exploring the phenomenology of the disaster response from a psychoanalytically informed intrapsychic viewpoint, a complementary team of Buffalo Creek researchers had begun investigating the same wealth of clinical data from a multivariant statistical perspective. Gleser, Green, and Winget (1981) reviewed the original reports generated by the UC teams of mental health professionals, along with reports on each survivor that had been generated by the psychiatrist for the defense. These became the data source for their empirical investigation into the effects of the dam collapse and flood on both the adult and child survivor populations.

Combining data from these two sources for the 381 Buffalo Creek adult survivors who had been assessed, and using the Psychiatric Evaluation Form to quantify the reports, Gleser et al. (1981) found symptoms of anxiety, depression, grief, apathy, sleep disturbance, and overall distress levels comparable to outpatient psychiatric patient norms among the survivors. Eighty percent of adult survivors were found to have some type of psychopathology. Investigators were also able to demonstrate the statistical relationship between the nature and severity of the disaster experience and individual psychopathology. Principal findings indicated that extent of bereavement (number and closeness of persons killed in the flood) was significantly predictive of the level of psychopathology two years after the flood. Extent of stressors experienced at the time of the flood (injury, threat to life, property loss) were also statistically predictive of two-year post-flood psychological adjustment.

The reports of the 207 assessed child and adolescent survivors were quantified in a similar manner as the adults. Findings indicated that they exhibited fewer symptoms of psychiatric impairment than did the adults. Approximately 20 percent of children had moderate to severe anxiety and 30 percent had depression and overall impairment. Statistically, there was a general tendency for the degree of pathology in children to be positively related to age, with older children exhibiting more distress than younger children. Levels of distress in children, particularly overall impairment and depression, were significantly correlated with their flood experience in a similar manner to adults. Gleser et al. (1981) were also able to demonstrate a statistical relationship between parents' and children's symptom distress scores.

Taken together, the publication of these earliest descriptions of the Buffalo Creek Syndrome from both clinical and empirical studies contributed significantly to the widespread acceptance that there was indeed a posttraumatic psychological syndrome. This body of work was frequently referenced by other disaster researchers and was influential in the introduction of Posttraumatic Stress Disorder (PTSD) as a discrete diagnostic category in the DSM-III (APA, 1980).

The empirically based branch of Buffalo Creek research for both the adult and child survivors continued into the second decade with the funding of two NIMH grants (Green, 1985, 1987). In each of these studies, the original reports from the clinicians for the litigants and the defense were used to establish a "probable" diagnosis of PTSD for that two-year investigation. This was necessary since the diagnosis of PTSD had not been formulated at the time of the original study, and yet the second decade investigation of both the children and adults was concerned with rates of recovery from PTSD from the first to the second decade.

In 1986, Green and her colleagues (Green et al., 1990) returned to Buffalo Creek and reinterviewed 120 of the 381 adult survivors who had been assessed originally, a figure representing

30 percent of the living members of that group. Using the Structured Clinical Interview for DSM-III (SCID), the diagnostic interview covering all Axis I diagnoses, 28 percent of survivors were found to have flood-related PTSD into the second decade. This represented a significant decline from the estimated 44 percent of survivors retrospectively assigned a PTSD diagnosis in the review of the two-year postflood assessments. Other measures of psychological functioning also showed a significant decline from the first to the second decade.

In 1989, the team led by Green (Green et al., 1994) again returned to the Buffalo Creek Valley to assess the status of the 207 originally studied children and adolescents who had moved on to young adulthood (17 to 32 years old). Ninety-nine such survivors were interviewed, again using the SCID as the basis of the diagnostic interview and a retrospective report review to determine "probable" PTSD in 1974. Results indicated that the rate of disaster-related PTSD in 1989 was 7 percent, down from a 1974 postflood rate of 32 percent. There were no age-related differences found, although all cases of persistent PTSD were women. As previously explained, it was this latest empirical study that then stimulated the further psychodynamic investigation concerning questions of meaning and adaptation, of which this current study is an outgrowth.

METHODOLOGY

The protocol for the videotaped interviews which compromise the database for this current study was developed to explore those questions of meaning and adaptation which the authors' prior study sought to investigate in "Portraits of Survival" (1993). The interview team of seven psychiatrists planned a psychodynamic interview format that permitted the interviewers sufficient latitude to follow the subjects' own associations while, at the same time, ensuring sufficient consistency amongst the interviews so that they could be compared for research purposes.[1] As had been the case with the original Buffalo Creek interviews, whenever possible these assessments were carried out in the subjects' own homes.

After an initial introduction including an explanation of the purpose of our investigation and its connection to prior UC studies, the beginning phase of the interview was left as unstructured as possible so that the subjects' memories of the flood and their spontaneous associations to these memories might lead to an understanding of the meaning of the flood experience to their subsequent lives. Following these initial accounts of the flood, we asked more specifically about their flood experience, including decisions made at the time and in the immediate aftermath, family responses, and flood-related dislocations. The subjects were then questioned about their postflood emotional development through adolescence and early adulthood, including the evolution of intimate relationships and careers. Although specific attention was then paid to their contemporary life situations and current symptoms of emotional problems, no attempt was made to comprehensively explore active PTSD symptomatology, as that had been the focus of the earlier SCID group level study. Inquiry was directed toward sleep problems, anxiety symptoms, depression, and substance abuse. In addition, the subjects were asked to describe a highly stressful life event that had occurred during the past few years and to compare this with the stress of the flood. Also elicited was a description of a recent hassle and how it was managed, recollections of dreams from the immediate postflood period and currently, and a drawing of their remembrance of the flood experience. Subjects had performed this latter activity during their childhood as part of the original lawsuit evaluation.

As reported in our prior study, the initial review of these tapes led us to explore the effect of the trauma on subsequent character development, which we eventually concluded was among the most

---

[1]All seven psychiatrists were University of Cincinnati, Department of Psychiatry faculty members. Four were child psychiatrists and six had been members of the original 1974 lawsuit assessment team.

important and persistent long-term effects on the child and adolescent survivors. Nevertheless, we were impressed as well that our interviews had elicited in a number of individuals symptoms of posttraumatic stress disorder that had not been reported during the earlier SCID interviews, as well as a number of seemingly trauma-related emotional symptoms that were not included in the DSM (at that time, DSM-III-R) criteria for PTSD.

As we began to study this latter finding in more depth, we became increasingly sensitive to the interview process itself, and the exploration of which features of that process had allowed these additional symptoms to emerge. Consequently, our research focus shifted to include more attention to the quality of the rapport, which had evolved between the interviewer and subject, and the affective states of each as the interview progressed and various content areas were explored. We began to take note of how the various interviewers dealt with resistances to communication and encouraged or impeded the subjects' recall and affective expression. Several clinicians who participated in the review of their own interviews were able to identify specific countertransferences that had impeded the subjects in elaborating on descriptions of prior and current distress. One member of our research team, who had also participated in the group level study, particularly noted how much more time was spent drawing the subjects out and getting them to elaborate their flood experience. One of the subjects contrasted the two research interviews as follows:

Subject (in describing the SCID interview): They didn't go specifically on just that one incident, the disaster. They did different categories. This digs deeper.
Interviewer: Would you answer differently now?
Subject: Yes, with this you have to sit and think about it. It digs up a lot of pain.

As we studied in more depth our subjects' behavior during the interview, we became aware of instances where symptoms of PTSD were verbally denied while simultaneously being enacted with the interviewer. Instances of avoidance and psychogenic amnesia (both PTSD C cluster symptoms) related to recall of specific horrors associated with the flood were noted, as was flatness of affect and melancholia, all possible symptoms of psychic numbing that had not been reported during the SCID interviews for these same subjects. In addition, several subjects exhibited a fixed stare in telling of the flood. This seemed to be a sign that the subjects were feeling as if the flood were recurring at the moment of the interview (a B cluster PTSD symptom). Also observed were instances where PTSD symptomatology had been displaced to other areas of concern where they were not recognized by the subject as flood-related and, therefore, had not been reported to the SCID interviewer. For instance, one woman denied hypervigilance (a D cluster symptom) related to the fear of recurring disaster, while later telling us that she worried constantly about her children's safety.

These observations, gleaned through our initial study of the process, as well as the content of our interviews, led us to evolve a protocol for the further review of our tapes. At least three research team members were present for every viewing and were initially "blind" as to earlier SCID findings related to the presence or absence of PTSD symptoms for each subject. At each point during the interview when a team member thought they had observed a flood-related symptom, the tape was stopped and the particular segment further reviewed until consensus was reached as to whether symptom criteria had been met. We then checked the SCID results to see if the symptom in question had been reported in the group level study. Flood-related symptoms that were not included in DSM-III-R criteria for PTSD were also described and discussed at length. Each videotape was reviewed twice in this manner, and at the conclusion, the SCID results were again checked to determine if the team had missed any PTSD symptomatology that had been reported to the SCID interviewers.

RESULTS

The videotaped clinical interviews of six subjects were reviewed in the manner described. Five subjects were found to evidence some symptoms of PTSD and of these five, four evidenced PTSD symptoms that had not been reported in the earlier SCID interview. Reciprocally, for two of the subjects, PTSD symptoms had been elicited by the SCID that were not discovered in the review of the clinical interview.

The central finding was that of a total of twenty-five PTSD symptoms for these six subjects elicited by the two methodologies combined, eighteen were elicited only by means of the clinical interview while three were elicited only by means of the SCID. The remaining four symptoms were discovered by both methodologies. Of the eighteen PTSD symptoms discovered exclusively by the clinical methodology, five were PTSD B cluster symptoms of "reexperience," nine were C cluster symptoms of "avoidance and numbing," and four were D cluster symptoms of "arousal."

Consistent with the research plan of this study, symptoms of PTSD were included as findings only when they could be definitively linked to the flood experience. In several instances, the research team chose not to include symptoms that were not sufficiently exact as to DSM PTSD symptom descriptions and/or not definitively flood-related. Thus, for example, several subjects, who in the clinical interview evidenced a restricted range of affect or signs of chronic depression, were not diagnosed as having C cluster symptoms of numbing because we could not determine for certain when, and in response to what, these symptoms had originated. This was particularly an issue with those subjects for whom there had been multiple subsequent traumas in the immediate aftermath of, and in the years following, the flood. Although some of these subjects displayed likely evidence of C cluster PTSD symptoms such as restricted affect, detachment, and diminished interests, these symptoms appeared to be related to the cumulative trauma experience and, therefore, were not included in the tally. Inevitably, such "telescoping" of the sequelae of early and subsequent trauma will prove a problem in a study attempting to assess the effects of a trauma so many years after the event.

An additional related diagnostic difficulty was encountered when there was evidence present in the interview for the likely displacement of a posttraumatic symptom to another situation.

Thus, one subject described a sense of alienation after the flood when so many valley residents moved away, and his sense of community was dramatically altered. Within a few years, this individual went on to work in the coal mines and was frequently on strike. Often, flood memories were evoked during his long hours on the picket line. In describing this experience, he again spontaneously referred to his sense of estrangement from other members of the community who were not on strike. Although we could not definitively describe this man's experience as a flood-related C cluster symptom of detachment and estrangement for inclusion in our findings, we strongly suspected that the current and earlier sense of estrangement were mutually reinforcing and, perhaps, even had taken on the permanence of a character trait.

In a similar vein, two-thirds of the subjects studied described flood-related symptomatology not included in the current DSM PTSD symptom survey. Several subjects displayed what appeared to be an "obsessive" sense of responsibility which clearly seemed to have originated with the flood experience. For one subject, this phenomenon took the form of anxious, hovering worry about the safety of children. For another it took the form of a more adaptive undoing with a wish to take care of children in order to give meaning to the horror of having witnessed the death of an infant in the flood waters. Another subject described feeling that she was living through her children to compensate for her childhood having been taken away by the flood. Survivor guilt appeared operative in the genesis of these and other symptoms that interfered with vitality and enjoyment of life.[2]

Other phenomena elicited by the clinical interview which seemed likely sequelae of the flood trauma, but not described in the DSM-PTSD nosology, included persistent rage toward the perpetrators of the flood, preoccupation with thoughts of death, counterphobic behavior in the face of current physical danger, and nostalgia for the valley and community to return to its pre-flood condition. These and other PTSD-associated symptoms

---

[2]Survivor guilt was not included in the DSM-III-R PTSD nosology but is included as an associated descriptive feature in DSM-IV.

seemed to have evolved into character traits that had altered these subjects' view of life and their place in it.

DISCUSSION

Our finding that two-thirds of our subjects displayed symptoms of PTSD that were not reported on prior SCID evaluation, and that 72 percent of the total PTSD symptoms present were uncovered only by means of the clinical interview, would appear to demonstrate a need for the inclusion of this methodology in the design of studies that intend to investigate the long-term effects of disaster on children and adolescents. The additional finding of a number of trauma-related symptoms not currently included in the diagnosis of PTSD raises the further question of the adequacy of current diagnostic criteria to comprehensively describe the long-term effects of disaster.

Our intention in raising these questions is not to debate the validity of quantitative, statistical versus clinical research methodologies, but to fill a gap created by the growing tendency to investigate the effects of disasters and trauma exclusively by statistical analysis of group level data generated by standardized interviews and surveys. The current research addressing this gap in our own Buffalo Creek findings is both ironic and fitting. It is ironic in that our colleagues in the earliest Buffalo Creek research helped to pioneer the group level statistical approach. The earliest such study was introduced by Gleser et al. (1981) as "probably the first large scale investigation of the long term effects of a disaster using quantitative data and sophisticated statistical methods of analysis . . . [filling] . . . the large gap in our understanding of the psychosocial sequelae of the disaster . . . [since] . . . many of the previous studies on disaster victims are merely clinical vignettes and impressions of material gleaned from extended observations and interviews" (p. 5). It is fitting in that this research group has consistently questioned the unexplained assumptions about trauma at a given time; PTSD did not exist when the group first found it.

Several other investigators have raised concerns about an exclusive reliance on standardized interviews, surveys, and group level data to assess the long-term consequences of disaster on children, and a tendency to discount or minimize the psychological sequelae of disaster in this population. In this regard, Anthony (1986) cautions that "those who study children 'macroscopically' and globally may tend to overlook microscopic psychological consequences" (p. 303). Sugar (1989) comments that "assessment of children in a disaster needs to be done on an individual basis along with evaluation of the family, since proxy questionnaires allow for distortions and denial" (p. 177). He further discusses the problem of countertransference in the treatment of child victims in the face of their intense anxiety, panic states, and abreactions. He comments as well on the paucity of detailed reports of individual therapy of disaster victims in the literature and the common assertion that disasters leave little longstanding emotional effect. Within our own study we noted instances of interviewer countertransference interferences with the exploration of trauma-related emotional effects. Although the argument might be advanced that only by means of standardized instruments might such interviewer bias be eliminated, the results of our current study raise serious concerns about the possible incompleteness of the results obtained when they are not balanced by more in-depth exploration. Additionally, the "halo effect" is a well-recognized source of countertransference even with standardized tests. We would suggest that it is only through the careful review of interviewer–subject interaction that countertransference distortion can be reliably detected.

A notable exception to the trend toward the exclusive reliance on standardized methodologies in exploring the impact of trauma on children is evidenced in the work of Terr (1979, 1983) with the Chowchilla kidnapping victims. In that instance clinical interviews were utilized to study a population of children over time. Her work has greatly expanded our understanding of the short- and long-term effects of trauma on children and has begun as well to define differentiated long-term effects for different varieties of traumas (1991). The work of Pynoos and Nader (1989), which is informed by a depth psychological intrapsychic perspective, is also important in this regard. They note, for example, that children exposed to disaster distort their distance from the scene, and that pictorial representations of the trauma include details which they omit in their response to verbal questions.

In further reviewing our own findings, we took particular note of the fact that C cluster DSM PTSD findings were overrepresented among those symptoms elicited by the clinical interview, but not by the SCID. In fact, of the ten C cluster symptoms reported by the two methodologies combined, nine were discovered by means of the clinical interview and only one by means of the SCID. These C cluster findings encompass negative symptomatology characterized by "avoidance and a numbing of general responsiveness" and include psychogenic amnesia, diminished interest, restricted affect, feelings of detachment, and a sense of a foreshortened future (APA, 1987). We hypothesize that it is with such negative symptoms that repression and other defensive activity are most at work. This would make it difficult for the subject to overtly acknowledge such symptoms in response to a directive yes/no question. The psychodynamic interview, on the other hand, which by its nature deals with resistances as they emerge in the clinical encounter, would be more likely to elicit such symptoms. We believe this finding to be of further significance in that it is specifically these negative symptoms that are most likely to evolve into long-term character traits when there is no opportunity for working through the acute aspects of the trauma. Such characterological effects were the predominant finding in our own report of the Buffalo Creek children (Honig et al., 1993) and harken back as well to Titchener and Kapp's (1976) original adult survivor study where they cautioned that the effects of the trauma may appear to disappear quickly if we are not alert to the subtle covering up behavior and characterological adaptations that protect the victims from otherwise overwhelming fears and helplessness.

Terr (1991) also places particular emphasis on the profound personality changes which often result from children's attempts to protect the psyche and preserve the self as part of their long-term adaptation to trauma. Among these effects she includes massive denial and psychic numbing which include "relative indifference to pain, lack of empathy, failure to define or acknowledge feelings, and absolute avoidance of psychological intimacy" (p. 16). Terr (1990) concludes that "fixing these character realignments following traumatic maladjustments is probably the most significant contribution a child psychiatrist can make to the traumatized child's future" (p. 303).

The psychological sequelae which Terr describes closely resemble the C cluster DSM PTSD symptoms. The problem of eliciting such symptoms by means of standardized interview techniques was recognized by the PTSD advisory committee for DSM-IV which noted the difficulty in operationalizing criteria for the assessment of denial symptoms such as psychogenic amnesia and a sense of a foreshortened future. In discussing this issue, Green (1993) comments:

The issue of the subject having to make the link between trauma and symptom him or herself is important. But it is also important to consider the issue of how certain criteria are operationalized both conceptually . . . and in terms of how questions are asked of research subjects . . . it is one thing for a clinician to listen to a patient for many hours and surmise that the person does not project him or herself in the future the way other patients do. It is quite another to devise a question that can assess this in one or two minutes in a standardized interview . . . [p. 95].

In this regard, we take note that although Green et al. (1994), in the seventeen-year follow-up of the children and adolescent survivors of Buffalo Creek by means of the standardized interview, found a decrease from the earlier study of this population in overall anxiety, belligerence, somatic concerns, and agitation, no decrease over time was discovered in the average depression rating. Here again, we would question whether in some subjects this finding of enduring depression might represent permanent character change wrought by the persistence of C cluster avoidant symptoms that had not been elicited by the PTSD/SCID interview for these same subjects.

Other investigators (Handford, Mayes, Mattison, Humphrey, Bagnato, Bixler, and Kayles, 1986) have noted the numerous methodologies utilized in child disaster studies, ranging from child observations and anecdotal reports, comprehensive interviews, interviews supplemented by projective testing or subjected to content analysis, questionnaires, standardized behavior rating scales, and self-report instruments. Although the comparison of studies is hampered by the lack of standardization, the wealth of information generated promises ultimately to lead to a better understanding of the long-term effects of trauma on children. Toward this goal we feel there is mounting evidence to suggest the need for a more comprehensive methodology which would include a clinical interview. In addition, diagnostic criteria for PTSD should be expanded to more comprehensively include expressions of trauma-induced character change.

CONCLUSION

In this study, through the review of the videotaped clinical interviews for six subjects, we found eighteen symptoms of PTSD that had not been elicited in a prior investigation utilizing the SCID. In addition, we noted trauma-induced character change as well as displacements and survivor guilt. These latter trauma effects are not included in current diagnostic categories, although they have affected the view of life and adaptation of the trauma victims.

To conclude this report, we will return briefly to that day of the "black water" in Buffalo Creek and the perspective of the inhabitants. For the individual, we imagine the first few moments of the incredible sight and overwhelming sound of the wall of water, the chaos, and the sense of the world ending. Then, after the escape to relative safety and in the long aftermath of emergency rebuilding, the larger world had not ended, but the smaller world of that valley nearly had. As the survivor learned of the devastation, the destruction, injury, and death, he or she felt connected to that as well as to the memory of the first few moments. The losses were numerous, so much that one felt strange if there were no personal ones. Something of the community, a large something, had vanished never to return. How could a child comprehend all of this? Not very well we imagine. Is that really so? It is our belief that all catastrophes to human beings are experienced in this way—sensibility crushed by unruly chaos and nearness of death followed by the indelible imprint of death, loss, and devastation to the surround (it stinks of mortality). This is followed by reorganization of the self, the family, the community and the economic, social, and political systems with varying degrees of completeness and flexibility for subsequent living.

The precise details of reorganization and recovery can be discovered and reported in various ways. We have used two fairly distinct, equally traditional methods employed in researching the child and adolescent inhabitants of the valley where the "black water" came down almost twenty-five years ago, to come to our current understanding of the children of Buffalo Creek. There are disasters to come, some with stultifying effects because of severity of trauma or lack of healing therapeutic response. Only through carefully designed studies capable of assessing the full breadth of the traumatic aftermath will we be able to better determine who among the victims are most in need of the therapeutic intervention that might prevent the all too frequent devastating consequences of trauma-wrought personality change. We hope this present study is a contribution in that direction.

REFERENCES

American Psychiatric Association (1980), *Diagnostic and Statistical Manual of Mental Disorders*, 3rd ed. (DSM-III). Washington, DC: American Psychiatric Press.
——(1987), *Diagnostic and Statistical Manual of Mental Disorders*, 3rd ed. rev. (DSM-III-R). Washington, DC: American Psychiatric Press.

Anthony, E. J. (1986), The response to overwhelming stress: Some introductory comments. *J. Amer. Acad. Child Psychiatry,* 25:299–305.

Gleser, G. C., Green, B. L., & Winget, C. N. (1978), Quantifying interview data on psychic impairment of disaster survivors. *J. Nerv. Ment. Dis.,* 166:209–216.

——— ——— ——— (1981), *Prolonged Psychosocial Effects of Disaster.* New York: Academic Press.

Green, B. L. (1985), Long term follow-up of disaster survivors. NIMH grant #ROI MH40401. (Available upon request from NIMH).

——— (1987), Children in disaster: Long term psychological consequences. NIMH grant #ROI MH 42644. (Available upon request from NIMH).

——— (1993), Disasters and posttraumatic stress disorder. In: *Posttraumatic Stress Disorder: DSM-IV and Beyond,* ed. J. Davidson & E. Foa. Washington, DC: American Psychiatric Press, pp. 75–97.

——— Grace, M. C., Vary, M. G., Kramer, T. L., Gleser, G. C., & Leonard, A. C. (1994), Children of disaster in the second decade: A 17-year follow-up of Buffalo Creek survivors. *J. Amer. Child Adol. Psychiatry,* 33:71–79.

——— Lindy, J. D., Grace, M. C., Gleser, G. C., Leonard, A. C. Korol, M. S., & Winget, C. (1990), Buffalo Creek survivors in the second decade. *Amer. J. Orthopsychiatry,* 60:40–54.

Handford, H. A., Mayes, S. D., Mattison, R. E., Humphrey II, F. J., Bagnato, S., Bixler, E. O., & Kayles, J. D. (1986), Child and parent reaction to the Three-Mile Island nuclear accident. *J. Amer. Acad. Child Psychiatry,* 25:346–356.

Honig, R. G., Grace, M. C., Lindy, J. D., Newman, C. J., & Titchener, J. L. (1993), Portraits of survival: A twenty-year follow-up of the children of Buffalo Creek. *The Psychoanalytic Study of the Child,* 48:327–355. New Haven, CT: Yale University Press.

Newman, C. J. (1976), Children of disaster. *Amer. J. Psychiatry,* 133:306–312.

Pynoos, R. S., & Nader, K. (1989), Children's memory and proximity to violence. *J. Amer. Acad. Child & Adol. Psychiatry,* 28:236–241.

Stern, G. M. (1976), *The Buffalo Creek Disaster: The Story of the Survivors' Unprecedented Lawsuit.* New York: Random House.

Sugar, M. (1989), Children in a disaster: An overview. *Child Psychiatry Hum. Dev.,* 19:175–177.

Terr, L. D. (1979), Children of Chowchilla. *The Psychoanalytic Study of the Child,* 34:547–550. New Haven, CT: Yale University Press.

——— (1983), Chowchilla revisited: The effects of psychic trauma four years after a school-bus kidnapping. *Amer. J. Psychiatry,* 140:1543–1550.

——— (1990), *Too Scared to Cry.* New York: Harper & Row.

——— (1991), Childhood traumas. *Amer. J. Psychiatry,* 148:10–20.

Titchener, J. L., & Kapp, F. T. (1976), Family and character change at Buffalo Creek. *Amer. J. Psychiatry,* 133:295–299.

12
Lethal Identity

Violence and Identity Formation

DAVID A. ROTHSTEIN, M.D.

EXPECTATIONS FOR THE POST COLD WAR WORLD

It has been said that it is very difficult to make predictions, especially about the future. At the turn of the century, there was widespread expectation that the millenium would be completed in an era of peace. Similarly, it was widely expected that the fall of communism and the end of the cold war would lead to an unprecedented period of peace and tranquility. Instead, the twentieth century turned out to be the most violent century in history, and the end of the cold war has not led to peace. Some have said the twentieth century began and ended with Sarejevo.

Cohen (1992) regards the end of communism as less important than the disintegration of multiethnic states. Woodrow Wilson's post-World War I reliance on the concept of national self-determination did not work out any better after World War II. The concept of national self-determination was flawed because it never made it possible to determine how large or small a group or territory would need to be to become a nation entitled to self-determination. It is possible that his father's Confederate sympathies during the Civil War influenced Woodrow Wilson in his formulation of the concept. Daniel Patrick Moynihan has described the flaws in the concept of self-determination (Moynihan, 1993), noting that the significance of ethnic conflict has been largely overlooked in the writing of twentieth century history.

WHY VIOLENCE?

Some time ago I put together a panel at an Annual Meeting of the American Society for Adolescent Psychiatry on the role of violence in identity formation, and published two papers on the role of violence, the military, and war in identity formation (Rothstein, 1975, 1983). I wrote about the particular appeal of violence and its frequent role in identity formation, particularly in adolescence, and not only in disturbed individuals, but also for the majority of those who make up the fabric of society. Violence plays a part in larger scale group and national identity, and there is an interplay between the violent solutions on an individual level and those on a larger scale social level. The violence inherent in socially approved solutions may foster the violence of disturbed individuals. More often, it "goes underground" in the solutions of the greater majority of the relatively "well-adjusted" individuals, but the solutions found by these individuals contribute to the eventual resurfacing of the violence on the larger scale social level, in particular in the form of war. War is not necessarily a part of basic human nature. It is a social institution perpetuated by social phenomena that interact with individual psychology, particularly in the crucial area of adolescent identity formation (Rothstein, 1983).

Horowitz (1985) has noted:

[A] group drive to obtain positive social identity by competition and comparison with other groups . . . quite apart from whether there is any rivalry for material rewards. Groups aim at distinguishing themselves from others on some positively valued dimension . . . [even when] experiments enabled them to do this by pursuing a course . . . that was not instrumentally "rational"—that is, it did not maximize profit, but it did maximize differentiation [p. 146].

As described by the Group for the Advancement of Psychiatry (1987):

Being one with the community confers great benefits, ranging from personal sustenance and even survival to participation in magnificent cultural achievement. But paradoxically, group-belonging can also lead to killing and to the destruction of culture in war . . . people experience their most intimate personal involvement in the nation's life in its most intense pitch . . . in war [p. 3].

The individual's ultimate identity depends on the modification, stabilization, and integration of earlier childhood relationships in the family and on a consequent ability to relate to, and identify with, groups in healthy and discriminating ways. The emotional roots of ethnicity lie in affects attached to it in all phases of life, but particularly those connected with very early life (Group for the Advancement of Psychiatry, 1987).

Volkan (1988) has described how this begins in early life. The individual externalizes and projects both undesirable as well as desirable aspects of himself or herself. Projecting the negative characteristics onto others, or onto institutions or symbols, provides obvious relief. Externalizing desired attributes allows them to be placed in safekeeping, deposited in the durable external reservoirs which these others, institutions or symbols, are hoped to represent. The next critical period is adolescence. During adolescence, ethnic and national identity become something for which one is willing to die. The need to have political enemies and allies results from our efforts to find a cohesive self and to form integrated representations of others.

In normal adolescence the loosening of ties to internalized self and object representations brings a mourning experience. . . . The adolescent then seeks new representations of self and object as replacement for what has been lost. As the adolescent's horizons expand beyond family and neighborhood, the world at large is observed from a new point of view. Familiar objects such as flag, food, language, and skin color continue to provide material for externalization, but now abstract conceptualizations infused with affect such as ethnicity appear . . . [as well as] other binding factors such as devotion to the same leader [Group for the Advancement of Psychiatry, 1987, pp. 50–51].

RESONANCES BETWEEN LEADERS AND FOLLOWERS

Binion (1976) quoted Hitler: "That is the miracle of our times: that you found me—among so many millions! And that I found you is Germany's fortune!" As I said in an earlier paper,

Whatever the psychological factors which led Hitler to develop in the way he did, the matter of understanding his personal development pales in comparison to the question of why the German people followed him. Leaders do govern by the consent of the governed. Hitler said that "what is essential will always be the inner accord between leader and multitude" (Binion, 1976) [Rothstein, 1983].

Zonis (1991) considered that leaders perform functions for followers. To help to regulate their self-esteem, individuals often select as self-objects, items of a public nature, such as specific persons, symbols, institutions, political systems, or ideas, which become part of their self-system. Such self-objects can be the president, the flag, military strength, national economic power, "standing tall," etc. The fate of these self-objects is crucial to the individual's self-esteem and feeling of well-being. The successful leader empathically recognizes these self-objects and husbands, nurtures, cares for, and even elevates the followers' self-objects. The leader makes him- or herself available as an object of identification and must withstand the pain of idealization. The particular personal characteristics of the leader interact with the contemporary historic events in determining how well the leader performs these functions for the followers.

CASE ILLUSTRATIONS

I will now describe some events in adolescence which illustrate and clarify how the processes which began in infancy and childhood are carried further in adolescence, and have an effect on the resonances between leaders and followers.

CASE 1. TOMMY

In his seventeenth summer, Tommy imagined into existence "The Royal United Kingdom Yacht Club," an imaginary English group of thirty vessels which he led as "Commodore, Duke of Carlton, Admiral of the White." He wrote a constitution for it prescribing that "The Commodore . . . shall preside over all the meetings of the Club, and no bill or resolution of any kind can pass into a law of the Club without his approval and signature. His veto makes a bill null and void, even if adopted unanimously by the Members" (Barber, 1972; Link, 1966).

Earlier in his teens, Tommy had begun to elaborate an imaginary world in which the British Navy played a significant part. He wrote out long detailed memoranda describing his fleets in minute detail. Tommy issued orders as commander; for example, as commander-in-chief, vice-admiral, duke, and "Vice-Admiral of the Red." His subcommanders and officers were usually friends or relatives, but some bore historical names. He created a fantasy world he could command and control.

Although an American, Tommy admired the English form of government. In an essay, he wrote of how much better off America would be with a parliamentary system of government and a sovereign, comparing the republican system unfavorably to the British one (Bragdon, 1967).

His academic record in college was undistinguished, but Tommy excelled in extemporaneous debate. He felt that the object of oratory "is persuasion and conviction—the control of other minds by a strange personal influence and power." He entered into a "solemn covenant" with a classmate that "we would acquire knowledge that we might have power; and that we would drill ourselves in the arts of persuasion . . . that we might have facility in leading others into our ways of thinking and enlisting them in our purposes" (George and George, 1964).

In college, "lacking a forum . . . [he] created one," the Liberal Debating Club, so that he could practice speaking before an imaginary House of Commons. In an undergraduate essay, he proposed "such changes in the structure of the government of the United States as would provide an outlet for his special talents and a field where he might realize his high ambitions." He was "irresistibly drawn to the debating societies of every university he attended. And . . . to the task of revising each club's constitution along the lines of the British parliamentary system" (Barber, 1972, p. 113).

About a year after graduation from college he left the name "Tommy" behind and became T. Woodrow Wilson or Woodrow Wilson (George and George, 1964; Freud and Bullitt, 1967; Barber, 1972). Tommy never did become an English admiral, but in real life he did go on to become Commander-in-Chief of the United States military and one of the nation's most successful presidents. He joined his country together with the British and others in the Great War and drafted a constitution for a world government, the League of Nations.

CASE 2: GEORGE (NOT HIS REAL NAME)

George first thought of the idea of starting a political party when he was 16. The name of the party was an acronym of the initials of the name he was using at the time. He prepared a notebook with a biographical sketch and planned to prepare membership cards. He said he got the idea for the organization from Germany and used variations of a swastika for its symbol. He decided to disband the party because people called him a Nazi.

Shortly afterwards he joined the U.S. military service. He decided that this would be a more positive identification and that by becoming a career serviceman his mother and relatives would not look down on him. He hoped that he might be able to some day meet the president and shake his hand. This hope was shattered when President John F. Kennedy was assassinated. Earlier he had written but not mailed a hostile letter to President Kennedy. He felt he could make up for the letter by going to the president's funeral. In order to explain his wish to his commander, he discussed his party activities. This precipitated further investigation of his background and led to his being discharged from the service.

A schizophrenic break followed during which he claimed to have paid Lee Harvey Oswald to assassinate the president and threatened to reinstitute his political organization. He allegedly said that he would consider the assassination of President Johnson to be necessary for the good of the country.

He was 18 years old when I examined him at the United States Medical Center for Federal Prisoners (MCFP) in Springfield, Missouri. I described his case in a paper entitled "Presidential Assassination Syndrome" (Rothstein, 1964).

CASE 3: EDGAR (NOT HIS REAL NAME)

Edgar was 19 years old when I examined him at the U.S. MCFP, although he claimed to be 24. He had daydreams of himself dressed as a cowboy, coming back to the institution, shooting all of the custodial officers, leaving a silver dollar near each body, and being nicknamed the "Silver Dollar Kid."

He had constructed about five additional years of his life in fantasy. During his first psychiatric examination at the MCFP, when, during the mental status part, I asked him who was president, he said he planned to assassinate the president as soon as he got out of prison because he (Edgar) was a socialist. He said he would get up on a roof and use a high-powered rifle with a silencer. By the end of that month someone did assassinate President Kennedy with a rifle.

It was felt that Edgar's fantasies and confusion about past events and his frequent but vague claims to be a socialist or communist resulted from a desire to associate himself with some group in order to establish an identity. He also spoke vaguely at times about belonging to some sort of secret organization. I also included his case in the paper on "Presidential Assassination Syndrome" (Rothstein, 1964).

CASE 4: FRED

The *Free Society*, the newspaper of a popular, dissident political cause carried the following warning: "ATTENTION. The attention of the comrades is called to another spy. . . . His demeanor is of the usual sort, pretending to be greatly interested in the cause, asking for names, or soliciting aid for acts of contemplated violence."

This referred to a man who, as Fred Nieman, had gone earlier to see the leader of one of the local groups following that cause and had met with a number of other party leaders in an attempt to be accepted as a member. "Far from accepting him, they were put off him by his queer manner and his ignorance of [their cause]" (Channing, 1902; Briggs, 1921; Donovan, 1964).

Fred had been a quiet, solitary child, increasingly bashful as he grew up. When he was 19 or 20, the workers at the wire mill where he worked went on strike for higher wages. The strike had a profound effect on him (Donovan, 1964). At about that time, he and his older brother began to rebel against the Catholic Church. At about age 21 he joined a local educational circle in which socialism and anarchism were enthusiastically discussed, began to have doubts about the American system of government, and resolved he would never vote again (Donovan, 1964).

Fred wanted to be associated with, and accepted by, the anarchists. "His desire to be an anarchist was so great that he thought he was one, and that was probably one of his delusions," although he apparently knew next to nothing about anarchist doctrine (Briggs, 1921). Fred's real name was Leon Czolgosz. He had been nicknamed "Niemand," meaning "nobody" by several German coworkers. He had clipped a newspaper account of the assassination of King Humbert I of Italy by an anarchist in July of 1900, read and reread it, and for weeks took it to bed every night. On Friday, September 6, 1901, five days after the item in *Free Society*, the anarchist newspaper, Czolgosz shot President William McKinley. Claiming to be an anarchist, Czolgosz said he had no grudge against the president, but that he did not believe in the republican form of government, in rulers of any kind, voting, marriage, or religion.

CASE 5: LEE

Lee wrote that he entered the U.S. Marine Corps at age 17 and that immediately after serving out his three years in the USMC he abandoned his American life to seek a new life in the U.S.S.R. "[F]ull of optimism and hope he stood in Red Square in the fall of 1959 vowing to see his chosen course through . . . " (Warren Commission Report, 1964).

He had begun to read Marx and Engels at age 15. He tried to join the Marines when he was 16 but the authorities did not believe his lie that he was 17. For the next year, "Lee lived for the time that he would become seventeen years old to join the Marines . . . " He studied the Marine Corps manual until "He knew it by heart" (Warren Commission Report, 1964; Warren Commission Meeting, 1964; Oswald, with Land and Land, 1967; Rothstein, 1964, 1966).

Six days after he became 17, Lee enlisted in the Marines. He became disillusioned with the Marines and the United States. Three months prior to his scheduled discharge, he requested transfer from active duty, ostensibly to care for his mother. Almost immediately he defected to the Soviet Union. Subsequently he became disillusioned with the Soviet Union. He was not quite 23 when he returned to the United States (Warren Commission Report, 1964).

After his return to the United States, he turned his hopes to Cuba and the Fair Play for Cuba Committee. However "his 'organization' [the New Orleans chapter of the FPCC] was a product of his imagination." Lee was the only member. The imaginary president was named A. J. Hidell, one of Lee's aliases.

Lee's "concepts and appreciation of Marxism were very superficial . . . he had no depth in his understanding of what Marxism was about" (Warren Commission Meeting, 1964). A reporter who had interviewed him in Moscow commented, "As he talked . . . I got the idea that he didn't know Marxism at all well" (Warren Commission Report, 1964).

On November 22, 1963, Lee Harvey Oswald assassinated President Kennedy.

CASE 6: NORBERT (NOT HIS REAL NAME)

During his adolescence Norbert noticed a change in his attitude toward public events. "The formerly patriotic little boy slowly came to detest all things of his native land.' He began to secretly cheer his country's defeats and humiliations. He read especially about one other country which he began to idealize. At age 15 he persuaded his parents to let him apply for an immigration visa to that country. Later, Norbert felt that he had been motivated by a growing idealization of an image which had grown out of innumerable books, magazines, movies, and newspapers which he had devoured.

During his earlier adolescence, he had developed an intense, deep friendship with a cousin of similar age. In order to signify their undying friendship they commissioned a jeweler to make two identical silver pins. They "secretly . . . plotted an elaborate scheme to run away from home altogether in order to live abroad."

Norbert's country had become totalitarian when he entered puberty. The country to which he "defected" was America. Norbert, now a psychoanalyst, indicated that in retrospect his reaction may seem to have been appropriate for a person belonging to a group which had become politically outcast, but looking back on it he knows he "was not motivated by any forebodings of future catastrophe," but instead by his idealization of America. He sees his action as having been determined more by his psychological need for an adolescent ideal than by a realistic interpretation of the political events in his country (Wolf, Gedo, and Terman, 1972).

Case 7: Ron

Ron wrote about the pleasures and pains of adolescence and about his ideals, ambitions, and dreams. He recalled the pleasures in his bodily sensations and the joy of mastering his athletic abilities. Although he was shy, he wanted to be a hero, to be stared at and talked about in the school hallways. He had an idea of what it was to be a hero: "Every Saturday afternoon we'd go down to the movies . . . and watch . . . war movies with John Wayne and Audie Murphy . . . Like Mickey Mantle and the fabulous New York Yankees, John Wayne . . . became one of my heroes."

But Ron and his friends were not mere passive observers: "We'd go home and make up movies like the ones we'd just seen. . . . We'd use our Christmas toys—the Matty Mattel machine guns and grenades, the little green plastic soldiers. . . . On Saturdays after the movies all the guys would go down to Sally's Woods. . . . We turned the woods into a battlefield. . . . "

They also made plans and formed a bond:

We studied the Marine Corps Guidebook and Richie brought over some beautiful pamphlets with very sharp-looking marines on the covers. We read them in my basement for hours and just as we dreamed of playing for the Yankees someday, we dreamed of becoming United States Marines and fighting our first war and we made a solemn promise that year that the day we turned seventeen we were both going down to the marine recruiter . . . and sign up for the United States Marine Corps [Kovic, 1976].

So Ron joined the marines. Of course, in reading his book, one already knows that Ron Kovic has been wounded in Vietnam and has become paraplegic.

Case 8: Sam (not his real name)

Sam remembered an intense relationship which he had with an older boy between the ages of 11 and 14. "We confided in one another. . . . We also engaged in various fantasy projects. We frequently pretended we were boy detectives, the heroes of an adventure story. . . . We conceived of a newspaper and even produced one copy . . . " At age 14, he and five friends formed a literary and philosophical society which met on Saturday afternoons to discuss philosophical, scientific, and aesthetic matters: "It was then that I began my reading of Freud and continued to cherish the wish that, impossible as it seemed, I might one day become an analyst." He did achieve the wish (Wolf et al., 1972).

CASE 9: WINSTON

Winston began school at age 7. "How I hated this school. . . . I counted the days and the hours to the end of every term, when I should return home . . . and range my soldiers in line of battle on the nursery floor" (W. S. Churchill, 1930). At age 13 he entered Harrow. His youthful patriotism was stirred by the Harrow school songs. Fifty years later, attending an annual singing of these school songs, he said with lively emotion, "Listening to those boys singing all those well-remembered songs I could see myself 50 years before singing with them those tales of great deeds and of great men and wondering with intensity how I could ever do something glorious for my country" (R. S. Churchill, 1966).

Winston joined the army class shortly before he was 15. When he was 16, he built a "den" at the family's new country house. With his brother Jack, his cousins, and other children on the estate, Winston built intricate fortifications around it, including a moat with a drawbridge, and a large homemade elastic catapult which propelled green apples. He went from drilling toy soldiers to drilling family members and friends (R. S. Churchill, 1966).

Winston was deeply interested in his work at Sandhurst (the Royal Military College). He later described his feelings:

It did seem such a pity . . . that the age of wars between civilized nations had come to an end forever. If it had only been 100 years earlier what splendid times we should have had! Fancy being nineteen in 1793 with more than twenty years of war against Napoleon in front of one! However, all that was finished . . . and now the world was growing so sensible and pacific—and so democratic too—the great days were over . . . [p. 44].

This complaint was destined to be cured, and all our requirements were to be met to the fullest extent. The danger . . . which in those days seemed so real of Liberal and democratic governments making war impossible was soon to be proved illusory . . . the South African War was to attain dimensions which fully satisfied the needs of our small army. And after that the deluge was still to come!" [W. S. Churchill, 1930, p. 75].

Winston Churchill wrote these last few paragraphs in 1930, as a fifty-six-year-old man, looking back over his earlier life. The major portion of his career might have been behind him. The deluge to which he referred was World War I. The impending deluge of World War II was still what he later described as a "Gathering Storm" (Churchill, 1948).

CASE 10: ADOLF

Adolf (Hitler, 1925) recalled that when his father retired, "It was at that time that the first ideals took shape in my breast." His father decided that Adolf should become a civil servant like he had been, but "my sympathies were in any case not in the direction of my father's career." Thus, at age 11, Adolf felt he was forced into "opposition" for the first time in his life. At age 12, he decided to become an artist. He later considered that two outstanding facts were particularly significant as resulting from this period of conflict with his father: "First, I became a nationalist. Second: I learned to understand and grasp the meaning of history."

He remembered his adolescence as "an especially painful process." When Adolf was 13, his father died. A few years later the death of his mother "put a sudden end to all my highflown plans." He later recalled, "In my hand a suitcase full of clothes and underwear; in my heart an indomitable will, I journeyed to Vienna. I, too, hoped to wrest from Fate what my father had accomplished fifty years before; I, too, wanted to become 'something.' . . . " He believed that at this time his "eyes were opened" to the two "menaces" of Marxism and Jewry. Vienna represented "the living memory of the saddest period of my life." The world picture and philosophy which took shape within him then became "the granite foundation for all my acts."

He recalled his reaction to the international climate of the time.

As a young scamp in my wild years, nothing had so grieved me as having been born at a time which obviously erected its Hall of Fame only to shopkeepers and government officials. The waves of historic events seemed to have grown so smooth that the future really seemed to belong only to the "peaceful contest of nations.". . . Why couldn't I have been born a hundred years earlier? Say at the time of the Wars of Liberation. . . . I . . . regarded the period of "law and order" ahead of me as a mean and undeserved trick of Fate. . . . "

The Boer War was like summer lightning to me. . . . The Russo-Japanese War found me considerably more mature. . . . Since then many years have passed, and what as a boy had seemed to me a lingering disease, I now felt to be the quiet before the storm. . . . And then the first mighty lightning flash struck the earth; the storm was unleashed and with the thunder of Heaven there mingled the roar of the World War batteries. . . . To me those hours seemed like a release from the painful feelings of my youth [Hitler, 1925].

Adolf wrote the above paragraphs in 1924 at age 35, at which time he was "nothing more than the organizer of street fights . . . the leader of a virtually non-existent party . . . " (Heiden, 1971). The translator notes that even in this work he was "fighting his persecutors, magnifying his person, creating a dream-world in which he can be an important figure" (Manheim, 1971).

Adolf had wished to start his own political party. Instead, shortly after World War I, he joined a small, newly formed, obscure, and weak party called the German Workers' party. He changed the party to meet his specifications. Shortly after joining, Adolf Hitler assumed leadership, expelled the founder, Anton Drexler, and changed the name to the National Socialist German Workers' party and eventually to the National Socialist, or Nazi, party (Hitler, 1925; Stevens, 1982).

CASE 11: JOHN

As a boy, John decided that he wanted to become a preacher. The family, living in the rural South of the United States, was very poor. He had no group with whom to practice preaching and no time off from his chores on the farm, such as taking care of the chickens. Therefore, John preached to the chickens. Later, with the help of a scholarship from the Reverend Martin Luther King, Jr., John went to college, and eventually was elected to the U.S. House of Representatives. Representative John Lewis gave a moving speech in Congress opposing beginning the air war against Iraq. He described his preaching to the chickens in a speech to the Annual Meeting of Physicians for Social Responsibility (Lewis, 1991).

THE PSEUDOCOMMUNITY

I will begin here by describing one of the characteristics which I found rather consistently in studying individuals who had threatened the president, or attempted, or succeeded, in assassinating a president (Rothstein, 1964, 1966, 1975, 1983). This characteristic, occurring during adolescence, consisted of membership or participation in an imaginary group, or an imaginary participation, or imaginary degree of participation, in an actual group. Upon further study, it became apparent that a very similar phenomenon could also be discerned in the adolescence of some leaders. I also noted that "The frequent interest in Russia, Communism, or Socialism seems to be conditioned by a desperate need to identify with at least any group, even a 'bad' group" (Rothstein, 1964). As a consultant to the Warren Commission and the National Commission on the Causes and Prevention of Violence, also known as the Eisenhower Commission, I noted that the threateners who espoused extremist political or ideological positions generally did not really understand the position and probably would have been disowned by the groups. They were really isolated but only wished to be part of a group and fantasied doing something spectacular to force recognition by the group (Warren Commission Meeting, 1964; Rothstein, 1968). The threateners' or assassins' expectations of approval from the group as a result of the act were sadly disappointed (Rothstein, 1973).

Weinstein and Lyerly (1969) studied threats and gestures of assassination as symbolic acts in the context of language and communication. They concluded that many subjects had "used the language of politics and other institutions to give them a sense of identity and relate themselves in what Cameron (1943a,b) has called a "pseudo-community." Such pseudocommunities were "the Kingdom of England and America" (for Richard Lawrence, who made an unsuccessful attempt to shoot President Andrew Jackson); the Confederacy (for John Wilkes Booth, who assassinated President Abraham Lincoln); the Stalwart faction of the Republican Party (for Charles Guiteau, who assassinated President James Garfield); the Anarchists (for Leon Czolgosz); and the Marxists (for Lee Harvey Oswald).

Cameron (1943a,b) introduced the concept of the pseudocommunity. He felt that the paranoid person is unable to get lasting reassurances from others to counteract his developing fear and distrust and creates a delusional pseudocommunity as an attempt at interpretation, anticipation, and validation of social behavior. Later, Cameron (1959a,b, 1967) also saw the pseudocommunity as a restitutive phenomenon, which re-establishes stable object relations on a delusional basis. He also pointed out that pseudocommunities are not necessarily confined to paranoid reactions, but can appear whenever delusional reconstructions include real as well as imaginary people.

There is one apparent difference between the concept of the pseudocommunity as introduced by Cameron (1943a,b) and the application of the concept by Weinstein and Lyerly (1969) and by me. For Cameron's paranoid patient, the pseudocommunity is hostile and destructive toward the patient; the patient is persecuted by his pseudocommunity. For Weinstein and Lyerly's and my subjects, the pseudocommunity is a group idealized in a positive way, which the subject wishes to join, not oppose. This difference may reflect whether the positive or the negative side of the subjects' ambivalence is predominant. The subjects I studied frequently shifted from idealizing one group to another. One subject had previously written a friendly, cordial letter to the president warning him not to take chances because there were dangerous persons around. Later he wrote a letter threatening the president.

However, I concluded that there was another important aspect involved. The pseudocommunity had many of the characteristics of what has been termed an academia.

THE ACADEMIA

Gedo and Wolf (1973) and Wolf et al. (1972) wrote about the creation of a private society, which they termed an academia, a special type of peer group involved with the reorganization of psychic structures that occurs during adolescence. Freud and his boyhood friend taught themselves Spanish in order to read Cervantes in the original. They "founded a strange scholarly society, the *Academia Castellana*" (Freud, 1960) and wrote letters to each other using the names of characters in one of Cervantes' *Exemplary Novels*, the *Colloquy of the Dogs*. Wolf et al. (1972) suggested that the essence of adolescence is the emergence of an inner necessity for new ideals, accompanied by opportunities encountered for such a transformation of the self. They saw the academia as a means utilized by the gifted individual whose change must be great. They noted that, for the majority of adolescents, heroes of sport or screen and occasionally historic figures usually provide the models for the new idealizations. Wolf et al. (1972) felt that examination of ready-made adolescent groups was unrevealing because the private meaning was largely unconscious.

However, utilizing the insights gained by these authors, I described how one can view such a ready-made organization as the army (or any military service) to see that it performs similar function for the ordinary person (Rothstein, 1983). Gedo and Wolf (1973) and Wolf et al. (1972) described the academia as affording protection for the expression of regressively reactivated grandiosity and to be helpful in the process of internalizing new structure.

I described the army and its activity, war, as performing a similar function. The process of removing old ideals and replacing them with new ones is intentionally fostered by the military. War is the perfect stage on which to act out archaic grandiosity—a domain in which it can be lived out (Rothstein, 1983).

Oliver Wendell Holmes recalled in a speech: "There is . . . a something more exalting, more ethereal, more word escaping than even our memories. . . . It is the fire of life . . . the men who have been soaked in a sea of death and who somehow have survived, have got something from it which has transfigured their world . . . " (Karsten, 1978). Gray (1970) noted that the experience of communal effort in battle has been for many veterans a high point in their lives, "the one great lyric passage in their lives." He described an expansion of the self: "We are able to disregard personal danger at such moments by transcending the self, by forgetting our separateness . . . the self is no longer important to the observer; it is absorbed into the objects with which it is concerned [resulting in an ecstatic experience], a state of being outside the self . . . breaking down the barriers of the self." Many cannot tolerate these extremes, but the experiences have a powerful effect on those who survive them, on others whom the survivors influence, and on institutions, such as the military, which perpetuate these traditions (Rothstein, 1983). I noted similar excitement displayed by some servicemen interviewed on television as they eagerly awaited the onset of fighting in Operation Desert Storm, and by some veterans reminiscing on television on the fiftieth anniversary of V-E Day about their experiences during World War II.

As I pointed out, "Unlike the academia . . . the army tends to transmit social values unchanged. In addition, the army influences the form of the academia for many creative individuals destined to become leaders. As a result, there is a natural resonance between the leaders and the population at large," which centers around war and violence (Rothstein, 1983). Both Woodrow Wilson and Winston Churchill utilized these phenomena to help them find an activity suited to their talents. On the other hand, the experiences of adolescence for Adolf Hitler had more of the quality of a pseudocommunity.

PRIVATE DETERMINANTS OF BEHAVIOR MANIFESTED IN PUBLIC AFFAIRS

I felt that the concept of the academia helped in understanding how private determinants of behavior come to be manifested in the world of public affairs. Adolescence is a crucial point in life when the individual withdraws his attachment from the family and redirects it to the outside world. The pseudocommunity is related to the academia, a normal phenomenon of adolescence. Just as the child not only projects negative aspects of him- or herself, but also positive aspects, the pseudocommunity, and especially the academia, can be a reservoir for positive as well as negative projections.

Some form of an academia or analogous phenomenon probably occurs to a greater or lesser extent in a majority of adolescents in our current culture. The means found to maintain narcissistic balance in the face of an inner necessity for new ideals, accompanied by opportunities for transformation of the self, can affect the resonances between leaders and followers. The academia plays a role in consolidating the differentiation between the self and the other on a societal as well as an individual level. Political events can call up remaining traces of phenomena which we have experienced to some degree during adolescence and which have been involved in our redirection from the family constellation to the outside world (Rothstein, 1975). There can be pseudocommunities whose meaning draws support from the needs of the leadership or the needs of substantial segments of society.

The United States essentially institutionalized a pseudocommunity with our cold war belief in monolithic international communism, which accepted the communist countries' assertions that they could attain a degree of economic success and a degree of cohesion and cooperation among themselves which had never been attainable by capitalist countries. Our fears of domestic communist subversion during the McCarthy era and some of our more recent fears of "crime," "drugs," and "Islamic fundamentalism" have characteristics of pseudocommunities.

ETHNIC AND NATIONALISTIC BREAKDOWN IN THE UNITED STATES

In addition to enlarging on the concept of the academia to apply it to the army, it appears that despite the reservations of Wolf et al. (1972), it may also be applicable to understanding the phenomena of cults and gangs. The apocalyptic end of the Branch Davidians has been compared to Masada. The Dead Sea sects, such as the Essenes, seem to have had much in common with modern cults (Group for the Advancement of Psychiatry, 1992). Perhaps further study can help in understanding the resurgence of religious fundamentalism. The militias, which have been in the news recently, appear to have qualities of pseudocommunities themselves, and, in turn, view the U.S. government and the United Nations as pseudocommunities.

Similarly, the quest for identity and self-esteem seems to relate to the role of violence in inner city youth gangs (Bing, 1991). While speaking with young men in a Gaza hospital and a rehabilitation center on the West Bank who had participated in the *intifada*, we were struck by the apparent similarity of individual dynamics to members of American inner city gangs. They were proud of their violent activities and of the resulting wounds. They defined their identity in this way.

The Chicago gang, the Blackstone Rangers, went on to change its name to the Black P-Stone Nation. A 1994 *Nightline* program focused on Louis Farrakhan's Nation of Islam and the anti-Semitic remarks made by his follower, Khalid Muhammad. Some of the discussion, particularly comments by Cornel West, professor of religion and director of the Afro-American studies program at Princeton, seemed to imply that such remarks were a misguided way of trying to bolster black identity (ABC News *Nightline*, 1994). On the right, groups are claiming to be establishing an "Aryan Nation," a "Christian Nation," or in other ways attempting to solidify their identity by establishing "pseudonations." A better understanding is necessary, not only to deal with specific gangs, "nations," etc., but also because there may be implications for the continuation or breakup of our own nation-state.

Moynihan (1993) says that "The point about the melting pot . . . is that it did not happen."

Schlesinger (1992) is worried by the lack of unifying American identity, and deplores the lack of a melting pot. He says, "The question poses itself: how to restore the balance between *unum* and *pluribus*."

PAST AND FUTURE

It would be interesting to know what may happen to these pseudonations. A detailed study of what has happened to similar pseudonations in the course of history would be enlightening but is beyond the scope of this paper. No doubt many pseudonations are not viable, and, like most random genetic mutations, they disappear. Others, however, may be like the occasional genetic mutations which power the process of evolution. Some of the pseudonations may turn out to be nascent nations, or develop into a distinct people. Two examples, the development of European nation states and the development of the Jewish people, may indicate a possible direction for study.

Freud (1930) said that "It is always possible to bind together a considerable number of people in love, so long as there are other people left over to receive the manifestations of their aggressiveness" (p. 114).

Volkan (1988) described the need to have enemies as well as allies. In fact, the need for an enemy other as a part of forming group identity and cohesiveness was noticed long ago. Gertz (1992) observed that Erasmus suggested using the Turks as the other. When Erasmus (1517) wrote "The Complaint of Peace," readers could look back on centuries of random, bloody slaughter and warfare between Christian nations of Europe. He suggested that "if, after all, the thirst for blood is so deeply ingrained in human nature that we can't endure without slaking it, wouldn't if be better to turn these fatal energies against the Turks?" and added that, "Since mutual charity does not bring Christians together, it's just possible that a common object of hatred may do so."

Suphi (1992) has described how the expulsion of the Jews from Spain in 1492 and the growing European hostility toward other unwanted elements in their societies, such as heretics, homosexuals, and lepers, played a part in the process of nation-building in European history. He believes that "there is real malignancy inherent in the development of nations in the West. During the evolution of nation states, people pushed away anything bad—like the Christians did with the Jews—in order to create for themselves an exclusive and pure national identity" (pp. 49–50).

But Jews also have a history of similar dynamics of nation building. I have described elsewhere how the *Haggadah,* which retells the Exodus of the Children of Israel from Egypt, portrays a process of nation building which needs the other (Rothstein, 1994a, 1995).

Before the story begins, there is a prayer, a part of which is, "Blessed are You, Lord our God, King of the Universe, who distinguishes between the sacred and the mundane, between light and darkness, between Israel and other nations. . . . You have distinguished and sanctified Israel with Your own holiness." The *Haggadah* tells how "We cried to the Lord . . . and the Lord heard our plea. . . . And God pulled us out of Egypt. . . . Has God ever tried to remove one nation from the midst of another nation . . . as the Lord your God did for you in Egypt . . . ? The Lord will give strength to His people; the Lord will bless His people with peace." But the Lord is requested to "Pour Your anger and Your wrath on the heathen nations that do not know You . . . " (Wiesel, 1993).

CONCLUSION

Looking back on history, at the unfulfilled expectations at the turn of the century that the twentieth century would be one of peace and democracy, the disillusioned hopes for a more tranquil world after the end of the cold war, the ethnic and racial violence, and the terrorism we now see, it is hard not to be pessimistic. But perhaps at this turn of the century—turn of the millenium—if we apply our reason, professional understanding, and human compassion, there can be cause for optimism. We now have amassed a significant body of information and experience in individual psychology and are developing an understanding of how to apply this on the larger scale level. Of course this can be abused and misapplied in a purposefully destructive way. I have described elsewhere how I believe that Radovan Karadzic, the leader of the Bosnian Serbs and a psychiatrist, and his psychiatric predecessor, Jovan Raskovic, may have done this (Rothstein, 1994a,b).

We are able to help our patients develop more adaptive psychological mechanisms once we understand the maladaptive means they have been using, once we and they understand what the symptoms have been doing *for* them, as well as *to* them, and recognize that these destructive and regressive mechanisms produce so many undesirable effects, eventually break down and undermine the very things they have been trying to support. So too, we should be able to help our species develop more adaptive mechanisms once we understand the maladaptive means it has been using. When we understand what these "symptoms" have been doing *for* us, as well as *to* us, and recognize how these destructive and regressive mechanisms produce so many undesirable effects, we hope that positive developments may overcome them.

An appreciation of how ethnic and national self-esteem have so often depended on violent and regressive mechanisms may allow us to find more adaptive ways to maintain ethnic and national self-esteem. When we understand how generation of an enemy has been such an effective and frequently used means of consolidating individual, group, ethnic, and national identity and cohesion, we are in a better position to develop less paranoid and destructive alternatives. Instead of focusing on, and nurturing, group, ethnic, and national self-objects with violent connotations, we can focus on, and nurture, others, such as an ideal of providing a better quality of life for all, excellent education, housing, nutrition, and health care for all. The end of the cold war is partly due to the fact that we have come to recognize that national security depends on such things as these more than it does on on military strength—perhaps so, too, can we come to recognize that this is also true for national self-esteem.

REFERENCES

ABC News *Nightline* (1994), *The Rift between Blacks and Jews*. March 3.
Barber, J. D. (1972), *The Presidential Character, Predicting Performance in the White House*. Englewood Cliffs, NJ: Prentice-Hall.
Bing, L. (1991), *Do or Die*. New York: HarperCollins.
Binion, R. (1976), *Hitler among the Germans*. New York: Elsevier.
Bragdon, H. W. (1967), *Woodrow Wilson: The Academic Years*. Cambridge, MA: Belknap Press/Harvard University Press.
Briggs, L. V. (1921), *The Manner of Man that Kills*. Boston: Gorham Press.
Cameron, N. (1943a), The paranoid pseudo-community. *Amer. J. Sociol.*, 49:32–38.
———— (1943b), The development of paranoid thinking. *Psychol. Rev.*, 50:219–233.
———— (1959a), The paranoid pseudo-community revisited. *Amer. J. Sociol.*, 65:52–58.
————(1959b), Paranoid conditions and paranoia. In: *American Handbook of Psychiatry*, Vol. 1, ed. S. Arieti. New York: Basic Books, pp. 508–539.
————(1967), Psychotic disorders. II: Paranoid reactions. In: *Comprehensive Textbook of Psychiatry*, ed. A. M. Freedman & H. I. Kaplan. Baltimore: Williams & Wilkins.
Channing, W. (1902), The mental status of Czolgosz, the assassin of President McKinley. *Amer. J. Insanity*, 59:233–278.
Churchill, R. S. (1966), *Winston S. Churchill*, Vol. 1, *Youth*. Boston: Houghton Mifflin.
Churchill, W. S. (1930), *My Early Life: A Roving Commission*. New York: Scribner's, 1958.
————(1948), *The Second World War: The Gathering Storm*. New York: Bantam Books, 1962.

Cohen, S. (1992), U.S. security in a separatist season. *Bull. Atomic Scientists,* 48:28–32.

Donovan, R. J. (1964), *The Assassins.* New York: Popular Library.

Erasmus, D. (1517), The complaint of peace. In: *The Praise of Folly and Other Writings,* ed., tr. R. M. Adams. New York: W. W. Norton, 1989.

Freud, E., Ed. (1960), Letters of Sigmund Freud (No. 37). New York: Basic Books, pp. 96–97.

Freud, S. (1930), Civilization and Its Discontents. *Standard Edition,* 21:57–145. London: Hogarth Press and the Institute of Psycho-Analysis, 1961.

———— Bullitt, W. C. (1967), *Thomas Woodrow Wilson: A Psychological Study.* Boston: Houghton Mifflin.

Gedo, J. E., & Wolf, E. S. (1973), Freud's novelas ejemplares. *Annual of Psychoanalysis,* 1:299–317. New York: International Universities Press.

George, A. L., & George, J. L. (1964), *Woodrow Wilson and Colonel House: A Personality Study.* New York: Dover.

Gertz, G. (1992), *Henry VIII: Humanism and Chivalry.* Typescript.

Gray, J. G. (1970), *The Warriors: Reflections on Men in Battle.* New York: Harper/Colophon.

Group for the Advancement of Psychiatry (1987), *Us and Them: The Psychology of Ethnonationalism,* Report No. 123. New York: Brunner/Mazel.

———— (1992), *Leaders and Followers: A Psychiatric Perspective on Religious Cults,* Report No. 132. Washington, DC: American Psychiatric Press.

Heiden, K. (1971), Introduction. In: A. Hitler, *Mein Kampf,* tr. R. Manheim. Boston: Houghton Mifflin.

Hitler, A. (1925), *Mein Kampf,* tr. R. Manheim. Boston: Houghton Mifflin, 1971.

Horowitz, D. L. (1985), *Ethnic Groups in Conflict.* Berkeley: University of California Press.

Karsten, P. (1978), *Soldiers and Society: The Effects of Military Service and War on American Life.* Westport, CT: Greenwood.

Kovic, R. (1976), *Born on the Fourth of July.* New York: Pocket Books.

Lewis, J. (1991), Speech to the Annual Meeting of Physicians for Social Responsibility, Atlanta, Georgia. March.

Link, A. S. (1966), *The Papers of Woodrow Wilson,* Vol. 1. Princeton, NJ: Princeton University Press.

Manheim, R., Tr. (1971). Translator's note. In: A. Hitler, *Mein Kampf.* Boston: Houghton Mifflin.

Moynihan, D. P. (1993), *Pandaemonium.* Oxford: Oxford University Press.

Oswald, R. L., with Land, M., & Land, B. (1967), *Lee: A Portrait of Lee Harvey Oswald by His Brother.* New York: Coward-McCann.

Rothstein, D. A. (1964), Presidential assassination syndrome. *Arch. Gen. Psychiatry,* 11:245–254.

———— (1966), Presidential assassination syndrome: II. Application to Lee Harvey Oswald. *Arch. Gen. Psychiatry,* 15:260–266.

———— (1968), Information and conclusions presented to the National Commission on the Causes and Prevention of Violence (Eisenhower Commission), Task Force on Political Assassination. Washington, DC, October 3.

————(1973), Reflections on a contagion of assassination. *Life-Threat. Behav.,* 3:105–130.

———(1975), On presidential assassination: The academia and the pseudo-community. *Adolescent Psychiatry*, 4:264–298. New York: Jason Aronson.

———(1983), The academia, the pseudo-community, and the army in the development of identity. *Adolescent Psychiatry*, 11:35–63. Chicago: University of Chicago Press.

———(Organizer, chair, and presenter, with J. Haas, A. Hussain, D. Horowitz, N. Itzkowitz, R. N. Lebow, J. Post, & N. Petkovic-Djordjevic (1994a), Breakup of multiethnic states in the nuclear age. Symposium Sponsored by the Committee on Psychological Aspects of Nuclear Issues, co-sponsored by the Committee on Human Rights, the Committee on International Abuse of Psychiatry, and the Area IV Council of the APA Assembly. American Psychiatric Association, 147th Annual Meeting, Philadelphia, Pennsylvania, May 24.

———(1994b), Paranoia and nationalism. Paper presented at International Society of Political Psychology, Seventeenth Annual Meeting, University of Santiago, Santiago de Compostela (La Coruna), Galicia, Spain, July 14.

———(1995), The discourse of the psyche: Identity formation and hate. Paper presented at the Midwest Modern Language Association, 37th Annual Convention, St. Louis, Missouri, November 2.

Schlesinger, A. M., Jr. (1992), *The Disuniting of America: Reflections on a Multicultural Society*. New York: W. W. Norton.

Stevens, W. L. (1982), *On Warfare*. Tape recorded supplement to book. Chicago: City College of Chicago.

Suphi, M. (1992), The expulsion of Safarad Jews: Regression in the development of modern society. *Mind & Human Interaction*, 4:40–51.

Volkan, V. (1988), *The Need to Have Enemies and Allies: From Clinical Practice to International Relationships*. Northvale, NJ: Jason Aronson.

Warren Commission Meeting (1964), *President's Commission on the Assassination of President Kennedy*. Report of Meeting of Members, Staff, & Psychiatrists, July 9, 1964. Unpublished transcript, pp. 7826–8071. Microfilm available from National Archives, Washington, DC.

Warren Commission Report (1964), *Report of the President's Commission on the Assassination of President Kennedy*. Washington, DC: U.S. Government Printing Office.

Weinstein, E. A., & Lyerly, O. G. (1969), Symbolic aspects of presidential assassination. *Psychiatry*, 32:1–11.

Wiesel, E. (1993), *A Passover Haggadah: As Commented upon by Elie Wiesel*. New York: Touchstone/Simon & Schuster.

Wolf, E. A., Gedo, J. E., & Terman, D. M. (1972), On the adolescent process as a transformation of the self. *J. Youth & Adolescence*, 1:257–272.

Zonis, M. (1991), Leadership and the world crisis. Paper presented at a Public Forum, Outreach Committee of the Institute for Psychoanalysis, Chicago, IL, March 11.

13

Xenophobia and Violence by Adolescent Skinheads

ANNETTE STREECK-FISCHER, M.D.

In recent years there has been an increase in extreme right wing attitudes amongst German adolescents, including xenophobia, accompanied by slogans supporting fascism and violence. Seen in the context of German history, these attitudes are frightening. In view of the activities of extreme right wing youths, we Germans again have to ask if the Nazi past is really gone, and particularly if psychoanalytic explanations of National Socialism that see its aftereffects as reaching into the third generation are sufficient to account for these adolescents.

Extreme right wing skinheads wear leather flying jackets, parachute boots, and close-cropped hair. They often carry weapons. They lie in wait for those they judge to be foreign or handicapped, or who appear to be politically motivated judging by their clothes and physical features. Skinhead violence is headlined in the news, as the following examples illustrate:

Two 17-year-old skinheads attacked 21-year-old B, kicked him, beat him up, and stabbed him fatally with a knife (*Göttinger Tageblatt,* January 2, 1991).

"I can't get rid of that hate anymore." Youth gangs play war, extreme rightists wage war on foreigners—thus fascism becomes an adventure playground for bored kids (*Die Zeit*, 1993, no. 1, p. 2).

Two skinheads with knives attacked a black Ghanaian in the Berlin S-Bahn (subway) and threw him off the train. He suffered a fracture at the base of the skull and had to have his left leg and two toes on the right foot amputated (*Die Zeit*, 1994, no. 44, p. 17).

Commuter trains in the suburbs of large German cities have become dangerous due to drunk teenage gangs. These groups show a frightening brutality. They are out to exterminate others (*Die Zeit*, 1994, no. 44, p. 22).

According to the German Office Responsible for Defending the Constitution, 70 percent of those who feel that strangers, foreigners, the handicapped, or dissidents are enemies, are adolescents, ages 13 to 20, 96 percent of whom are male. Therefore, one can assume that processes occur in adolescence which make teenagers susceptible to ideologies that promote hostility toward foreigners and others they view as "enemies." In this paper I wish to suggest that specific factors involving adolescence, personality, and culture may lead to xenophobia and violence.

LITERATURE REVIEW

Extreme right wing attitudes are founded on two basic ideas which are contrary to the values of democratic societies, one of which is that people are unequal. This is their core philosophy of life (Heitmeyer, 1987, p. 16), and along with it go nationalism, a grandiose self, racist views, xenophobia, a catalog of worthy and unworthy lives, emphasis on might equals right, and a totalitarian understanding of norms that excludes those who are different. The other basic idea is that of force, which the right wing extremists use as a central mechanism for regulating conditions and conflicts in society. Various explanations have been found for extreme right actions by adolescents, especially from sociological and pedagogical slants (Heitmeyer, 1987, p. 31; 1989). However, there are only a few psychoanalytic explanations of today's extreme right wing behavior of youths in Germany. Here it is necessary to fall back on explanations which are especially valid for reappraising the German Nazi past.[1]

Lowenfeld (1978) explained the significant rise of fascist ideologies in 1935 as due to the collapse of capitalism and its associated social and spiritual values. In times of catastrophes such as those, it is easy for a turn to the irrational to set in (p. 566). A leader-focused ideology, such as fascism, grows in strength as a result of reality disappointments and individuals ceasing to think in a reality-oriented manner, and regressing to earlier stages of development. Lowenfeld (1978, p. 572) feels that the mechanism of identification, of becoming more like and at one with the ideal or the leader ("the aggressor—my completion"), a mechanism which also serves to cope with the Oedipus situation, plays an important role in increasing self-worth.

Parin (1978) emphasized that an unstable sense of self-worth is especially susceptible to ideologies of power and to those who propagate ideas that people are unequal. Hochheimer (1962–1963) speaks of a "prediscouraged ego" (p. 489), which was denied the necessary narcissistic support from the social environment. Hacker (1990) described ten categories of the fascist syndrome, among which are maximizing inequality, the right of the stronger, irrationality, standardization, violence, and terror, which are legitimized by the fascist ideology.

In most publications (Lowenfeld, 1937; Adorno, 1951; Hochheimer, 1962–1963; Mitscherlich, 1970; Müller-Braunschweig, 1985), the origins of the extreme right and its xenophobic attitude are examined on a societal level, but adolescence and the biographical background of the youths of the extreme right are not considered. Eissler (1968, p. 457; tr. by author of this article)

---

[1] In older psychoanalytic concepts of adolescent development there is a tendency to pathologize this period. Viewing enhanced adolescent narcissism separately from the development of object relations has especially contributed to the confusion (see Ziehe, 1975).

discusses the adolescent's modes of reaction which are threatened by narcissistic emptying because of continual traumatizations, and states, "The only accessible source of lifesaving narcissistic refilling . . . was the narcissism of the controller of power and the way to utilize this source was identification." Winnicott (1965) mentions: "At present there really is a threat and the worst, which the tendency of today's adolescents to form violent groups could lead to, would be the start of a movement comparable to the beginning of the Nazi period. At the time Hitler solved the problem of the adolescents overnight by offering them the role of superego in society" (p. 203; tr. by author).

As a therapist I have seen youths from the extreme right who are openly militant. Usually people who suffer from their environment and are full of protest and resentment against society, do not come to psychotherapy and psychoanalytic institutions. They do not express their conflicts internally or intrapsychically, but externally, interpersonally, and socially. To my surprise some extreme right wing youths (usually after being urged by their parents) take advantage of therapeutic institutions at least temporarily, and this has encouraged me to investigate the psychic, social, and developmental conditions of these youths.

MALE ADOLESCENTS

Psychobiological maturational processes, and the beginning of separation from the parents during adolescence, lead to characteristic changes in the relationships of youths to themselves and their environment. When confronted with the feeling of being a stranger to oneself and to others, and being unable to use coping strategies from childhood, a crisis may develop which destabilizes the individual's self-system (Streeck-Fischer, 1994c).

The temporary phase of increased narcissism in adolescence results from experiencing the "developmental lag: the body has

changed, but the mind has not been able to keep up" (Giovacchini, 1978, p. 325). The increased transitional narcissism resulting from the physical and affective–cognitive changes is an
Achilles' heel of adolescence (Sarnoff, 1987, p. 37). Especially in
situations of insult and conflict, adolescents resort to self-percep-
tions in which they are great, irresistible, and capable of doing
anything, or they tend to imagine themselves as being totally incapable in reality, but particularly in fantasy. More complex perceptions and attitudes can be lost due to a partially weakened
perception of reality. Hartmann (1927) speaks of the capability
of checking reality and of the ego becoming labile. As a result
of transitional regression due to heightened self-cathexis and an
increase in drive pressure in adolescence, self and object differentiation can be minimized. The more the parents attack, the more
regression is required. Often, however, self and object representations remain as an internal frame of reference.

Male adolescents often resort to a transient narcissistic stabilization with an aggrandized self. This is a product of the fusion
of real and ideal pictures of themselves and of idealized objects
(Kernberg, 1975). This can be seen in the bragging and arrogant
behavior of some male adolescents. At the same time they do not
perceive others accurately and devalue them in an attempt to
make them less threatening. Unpleasant parts of the self are denied or projected onto others, who are then despised or attacked.
Introspection, which would lead to confrontation with one's own
inadequacies, is more often avoided by these adolescents. Inner
conflicts are externalized and acted out. The site of encountering
and analyzing oneself is more likely on the outside, either in
school or in the overall social environment (Fend, 1990). Narcissistic self-aggrandizement is accompanied by grandiose fantasies,
which compensate for the inadequacy experienced in this period
and which support the self-system. They often have a supportive
effect as a developmental program in growing up (Chasseguet-
Smirgel, 1975) by promoting steps in development which decrease the distance between one's ideal self and others, and the
real possibilities. Other stabilizers are good self, object, or identity

supports (e.g., particular heroes, movie characters, and adolescent-specific clothing accessories). Fusion experiences with objects of narcissistically increased status are sought in an effort to help overcome one's own inadequacies.

For example, teenager A has grandiose fantasies of being a famous scholar who provides knowledge to the military leadership during World War II. As Goering's deputy he saves Germany and establishes a German empire. After the death of Hitler and Goering he becomes their successor. "The world is saved by me." This fantasy is in total contrast to his current, desolate living conditions.

FEMALE ADOLESCENTS

In contrast, female adolescents tend toward narcissistic stabilization of a dissociated type associated with self-devaluation and splitting of ideal self and ideal object aspects in daydreams, fantasies of grandeur and rescue. They turn to the inside with withdrawal, depressive reactions, and preoccupation with their own bodies. This is often seen in female adolescents in connection with the narcissistic reaction. Therefore, as long as they do not identify themselves with males, female adolescents are less prone to orient themselves to an ideology, which supports stabilization of a grandiose self with an inherent phallic cult and counteracts fears of self-disintegration and castration fears (see below). Rather, female adolescents tend to subject themselves to destructive conditions as victims of others, usually males, who violate them.

ADOLESCENT PROCESSES AND THE EXTREME RIGHT

With increasing separation from the parents, adolescents may temporarily lose important controls on their behavior, parental guidance, and lose track of traditional values (Jacobson, 1964). Peers now become the prime external source of self-esteem, as parents had been in the past. Adolescents search for a feeling of oneness, or for a world of divided meanings (Emde, 1984) in their peer group. Until the end of latency this feeling of oneness still referred to the family. However, the peer group now serves as a bridge and a transition during the separation–individuation phase and offers relative support and values as long as the connection to the parents is not lost. As a field for experiments or an "autoplastic milieu" (Blos, 1976) it then has a supportive effect on development. If relations to the parents are broken off, then the group becomes a new family. As a consequence of regressive processes the realization of an infantile rescue fantasy (Lowenfeld, 1978) is sought in the peer group. Rescue fantasies, like the wish to rescue one's nation (Germany symbolizing the "maternal object"), may be understood as attempts to cope with infantile trauma. Adolescents with similar wishes are compulsively driven to repeatedly reexperience infantile rescue fantasy in sects or terrorist groups (Lowenfeld, 1978, p. 153). These subcultural groups often have a damaging effect on the personality development of the adolescent and adverse dedifferentiating effects on the personality as well (e.g., by means of narrow-minded verbal barbs that induce an extreme polarization between "good" peer group versus "bad" society). Certain accessories, such as a punk hairstyle, a Palestinian scarf, or a skating jacket further encourage feelings of oneness with a certain peer group and secure one's place in it.

Insecurities concerning sexual identity and masculinity lead to tests of courage and hyperphallic actions. In accordance with the "physiological" readiness of adolescents to think and perceive in contrasts, strength, toughness, and greatness are attributed to masculinity, whereas femininity is viewed as weakness, incapability, and cowardice. In order to elude the regressive suctionlike force of the early mother, which is significantly stronger for male than for female adolescents, cults and ideals of masculinity compensate against regressive fantasies, desires, and fears of castration (Gilmore, 1991).

The so-called "cold cultures" (Levi-Strauss, 1973) deal with the surging drive impulses in adolescence with rites of initiation which partly remind one of torture methods. These rites carry out tradition with force. Processes which could lead to cultural change are frozen. Therefore, social order and roles remain predetermined. In our so-called "hot culture," adolescence is viewed as a motor of social change (Erdheim, 1984). The process of adolescence, though, is increasingly characterized by deritualization and detraditionalization. The resulting individuation of one's own development often overtaxes adolescents and leads them into more isolation and alienation (Heitmeyer, 1992). From this perspective youth cults seem to be attempts to find security with the help of counterritualizations. Instead of progressive coping, regressive patterns become significant.

Central childhood conflicts influence all life phases as repetitions. For some adolescents the degree of neurotic disorder or trauma from early childhood determines whether infantile conflicts are repeated, or new experiences or creative coping are possible. For other teenagers their current conditions play a role, which can then become a "second chance" (Eissler, 1968) if the parents and other adults are available for discussions, identifications, and new experiences, and if the affective–cognitive structures (Piaget and Inhelder, 1977), which have now been developed, make progressive solutions possible. Thus, a vocational perspective as a developmental pattern offers the adolescent the possibility of coping with these central infantile conflicts, between progressive striving and regressive desires, with compromise formation. However, if the youth is not able to carry out his previously unmastered preoedipal and oedipal conflicts in dealing with his parents and other adults (which would enable him to accept real parental and societal contradictions), these conflicts are carried out on the threshold between family and society. Any deplorable state of affairs or political conditions can now be transferred in general to society. Transforming concrete experiences into political philosophies is not unusual for adolescents (Heitmeyer, 1988). Political publications are especially dangerous, if a kind of "Nazi milieu" exists in the family, whether Nazi ideologies are handed down, or whether in a fortresslike family intense hostility is demonstrated toward strangers, or whether the adolescent is seen as a failure by, and has always had the position of, the "hostile foreigner" in the family (Streeck-Fischer, 1994b).

XENOPHOBIA AS A FORM OF SELF-STABILIZATION WHEN THE SELF IS THREATENED

When youths are subjected to continuous trauma the developmental tasks of adolescence can become overwhelming. Adolescent skinheads with whom I have worked psychoanalytically, show a number of traumas. They are insufficiently bonded to unreliable, partly rejecting, inadequate mothers, or given up to foster care or adoption. The homes are mostly broken. The fathers remained absent, weak, and/or arbitrary, violent, and often devalued as alcoholics. In school, they do not achieve the goals set by themselves or their families due to learning deficiencies and aggressive, restless behavior. As troublemakers and outsiders they have experienced rejection by their teachers and classmates. Though they may be above average in intelligence, they have continual experiences of being inadequate and incapable. Leaving school early, or being demoted to lower level schools, has helped propel them toward their future life situation.

For youths who lack family ties and support, and who have continuously been denied appropriate narcissistic gratification and possibilities for identification and self-fulfillment, the tasks of adolescence pose a long-term crisis. When they are confronted with their inadequacies and insufficiencies, these adolescents rationalize and try to put the various narcissistic insults into relative perspective (Streeck-Fischer, 1992). Connecting themselves to extreme right groups offers them several stabilizing factors:

1. The right-wing group becomes a substitute family when relationships to the family and society are insufficient, or have been

broken off. The peer group (and within this group other adolescents with leader functions) takes over parental functions. The peer group then is not just a temporary place on the way to separation, but becomes the new family, and the path to individuation is blocked. The newfound comradeship makes up for the overwhelming feelings of loneliness many of these adolescents experience. The culture of violence in the skinhead scene damages the often traumatized adolescents in many ways. It is a scene of action which is attractive for teenagers with little education and low aspirations for the future. Openly destructive coping strategies are sought to overcome feelings of paralysis, powerlessness, and emptiness. The newfound comradeship offsets the experience of loneliness. The crisis of an insecure future is temporarily solved with clear defining principles.

One adolescent said: "You get a great feeling of power when a large a group of us runs down the street. Nobody dares to bother you, to touch you, even the police have respect for us. Besides, you get an awful lot of attention. People notice us. If we didn't look like this, or behave this way nobody would notice us" (Reimnitz, 1989, p. 184).

2. Becoming involved with racist ideology inflates the individual's own self by status enhancement with the fact that one is of German nationality by birth, along with the notion of being superior due to being a male. This tends to reduce the narcissistic insult felt up to that point. The ideology takes on a soothing, filling function for the damaged and threatened self (Morgenthaler, 1974). In the oneness with the ideology, which devalues and dehumanizes certain strangers, one's own deficiencies are defended against, externalized, and projected on strangers who are then rejected. Fantasies of grandeur, which served as compensation for one's own deficiencies, seem to be able to be realized instantly. As rescuers, custodians of the law, and protectors of the environment for this "threatened nation," they feel, to quote from a song by the band *Störkraft*, "We are the power which makes Germany clean." Increased self-esteem and narcissistic gratification are thus experienced. By fighting for the "threatened nation" which is idealized as an absolutely good object, their own threatened self is protected.

3. Self-hate is converted into hatred of strangers. One's own deficiencies and inadequacies—the hated parts of one's self—are projected on the stranger, the foreigner, and attacked in him. The hate is directed at someone who supposedly threatens the substance of the self. The enemy-other is needed to stabilize one's self in a symbiosis of opponents. The adversaries become locked in a permanent dance (Stein, 1990, p. 71). It is an entanglement in which the other experiences what is meant for oneself. Unbearable conflicts, impulses which are defended against, destructiveness, and self-hate are projected onto the chosen enemy, who becomes the target of hostility.

4. Uniforms are an expression of increasing conformity and deindividuation. Skinheads dress in a paramilitary style, with a mixture of exaggerated masculinity, toughness, and brutality. A regressive process is induced by all of them donning the same type of flying jackets and parachute boots, adorning themselves with tattoos symbolizing membership in the group, and listening to and singing fighting songs. This leads to conformity in thinking, feeling, and acting with noticeably primitive and angry ideas regarding the enemy-other (Hacker, 1990). The outward conformity corresponds to regression to early introjects (which are reactivated in the violent milieu) and which demand unconditional acceptance and submission in dangerous situations.

The ideology of the extreme right offers a substitute masculine identity in a phallic cult by exhibiting a mixture of exaggerated masculinity and toughness by which the deep feelings of inferiority and castration fears are overcome (Mitscherlich-Nielsen, 1983). A narcissistic desire for aggression serves as a substitute or compensation for unattainable sexual satisfaction after continual humiliations and renunciations (Shatan, 1981). Their sexuality, which has not been integrated yet in connection with an insecure sexual identity, is perverted into aggression and readiness for violence. To be ready for a fight and to be brutal, then become highly valued signs of masculinity and bravery. They are an expression of images of masculinity which recall societies at war and promises of heroism.

"When I'm 18 I want to shoot everybody and myself because I hate myself and will never have a girl friend," said S. Lust for violence becomes a substitute gratification, which, like any other addiction, is connected with dose increases. Eroticizing violence fosters the fighting addiction (Shatan, 1983).

CASE ILLUSTRATIONS

CASE 1

D, a 16-year-old skinhead, came to inpatient psychotherapy at the instigation of his father and stepmother. He had been living in a garden shed since his family had banished him from the home. After several school expulsions and quitting on-the-job training he joined a group of xenophobic, extreme right wing teenagers. To a certain extent he felt accepted there. As an outsider and a troublemaker he had experienced rejection everywhere, at home, school, and work. In the group he finally found friends, and by joining in violent group actions against foreigners he felt his status had been enhanced.

He wanted psychotherapy because his uncontrolled outbursts of anger frightened him, since he then became very cold and was afraid he could kill someone. He appeared full of despair and wanted to do everything possible in order to find a way out of his current condition. According to clinical diagnostic criteria, D had a borderline personality disorder (Internat. Klassif. Psychischer 1993 (ICD 10): F 60.31, F 91.1). The deficiency in his early mother–child relationship had led to deep disturbances in his ego organization and his self-system. Due to his relationships being on a part object level he was unable to integrate contradictory aspects of himself and others, and was in a disturbed, ambivalent state. Intimacy was dangerous for him, since it held the threat of regressive fusion, as was being alone, since that confronted him with unbearable feelings of emptiness and tension.

CASE 2

Although above average in IQ, M did not do well at school because of his aggressive–provocative behavior and a serious attention deficit hyperactivity disorder (ICD: F 90.1). He was expelled from upper-level high school. For disciplinary reasons he changed schools six times within two years, and finally ended up in the lowest level of high school. Here he joined the extreme right teenagers. At the instigation of his mother and stepfather he came to inpatient psychotherapy.

The mother of illegitimate, 15-year-old M remembered him as a child who was always difficult to control, restless and aggressive. He became especially difficult after his mother married, when he was 3 years old. In kindergarten, he was rejected by the group because of his misbehavior. In school, he always remained an outsider due to his distancing, aggressive, and provocative behavior. He was overtaxed by the academic and social requirements, and was an unbearable troublemaker with unsatisfactory grades. The family atmosphere was characterized by continual, severe, and sometimes physical arguments in which M was the center. He agreed to inpatient psychotherapy, superficially, to gain some distance from the unbearable conditions at home. M showed a strong tendency to avoid reality, and during his psychotherapy refused to see himself as someone who, because of his bad experiences, still had problems. On the whole, he seemed confused, without insight, like a stranger who was neither able to cope with himself nor his environment. He seemed to be armored, walled off, and cut off. Only with his skinhead group did he find the recognition and perspectives that he was seeking. Here he felt that he belonged with like-minded youth who projected everything bad to people whom they regarded as socially inferior, different, branded as bad, and thereby felt his status enhanced.

THE DEVELOPMENT OF THE PROPENSITY
TO VIOLENCE BY ADOLESCENT SKINHEADS

Shatan (1983) described processes for the militarization of male adolescents, which are comparable to the development of adolescent skinheads. The uprooting of the individual is followed by his dehumanization and the development of a paranoid fighting attitude including erotizing violence (Shatan, 1983). It is a deadly dance, which explains how a readiness for xenophobia and violence is aroused. Stein (1990) called the hostile entanglements of two nations which lead to war a "deadly dance." In my application of the phrase "a deadly dance," I describe a group process, in which the consequences are dangerous regression in thinking, feeling, and acting, and which lead to more primitive personality functioning. Such changes in personality function could often be observed during inpatient psychotherapy of adolescent skinheads. These group processes can be transferred to the formation of youth gangs. The "deadly dance" (Streeck-Fischer, 1994a) proceeds in the following steps

1. Loneliness, loss of perspective, and existential questions lead to a sense of a threatened self, connected with a severe narcissistic crisis. These conditions prepare the way for the individual to step into the skinhead scene. External circumstances are made responsible for one's unbearable and disastrous life situation. These youths increasingly tend to behave in destructive and illegal ways, which is a consequence of the inner and outer existential threat. In the inpatient setting, the malignant group processes, with actions which violate the boundaries, begin in the form of disregarding rules and deliberate provocations.
2. Regressive processes are set off in the group. Ambivalence toward strangers is lost, and an old/new enemy with a black or white status concept develops with delusional reality, misjudgment, and projections.[2] The threat which the individual originally felt is now transferred to the community which he feels

---

[2] *The old enemy concept* refers to the fact that every society (just as every individual with his or her family) historically has handed down certain concepts of an "enemy."

the selected "enemy" threatens to destroy. In the group, one's own existence is elevated, and together with others, a powerful, group-centered, aggrandized self develops. This fused group formation, which is directed against outside enemies, is a result of a regressive personality restructuring at a borderline level. While they are inpatients, such group members may put counselors in the role of the bad persecutory objects.

3. The selected enemy is dehumanized. Dissidents (e.g., the teachers) are dehumanized by distortions and myths, or they are viewed as filthy vermin or degraded to loathesome, perverse beings. When the enemy loses all human dignity then he can also be crushed.

4. Under the influence of alcohol and in a state of paranoid misperception of reality, with no inhibition of hate and destructive impulses, violence breaks out. To abuse the other, the chosen enemy, and see him bleed or destroyed serves to repair a damaged self, a self which was provided by the group, and magically attached to the country and the nation. Adolescents whose identity has been damaged by cumulative traumas and social ostracism tend to project onto such an enemy. The more threatened they feel the more delusional they become. The resulting dehumanization of the enemy object and violence derive from their previously experienced social and affective death.

In the background of their premorbid structures these adolescents experience foreigners in Germany as intruders into extended areas of themselves and the group. They try to use violence to reconstruct their own borders and cleanse their life spheres. The acts of violence are merely the last step in a long, disastrous development, which ultimately leads to a "deadly dance."

Empirical studies (e.g., Heitmeyer, 1992; Wellmer, 1995) substantiate the living and social conditions of adolescent skinheads as described here. In particular, negative perspectives for the future have adverse effects on adolescents' social development. Heitmeyer (1992) observes an increase of instrumentalization, which leads to objectification and depersonalization of, and an indifference to, human beings in capitalistic societies. Adolescents react very sensitively to such processes.

A society which shuts out from its institutions adolescents who are difficult, aggressive, restless, and have learning difficulties, leaves them without any hope for self-realization and brings forth youths who seek fulfillment in violence against, and destruction of, still weaker and similarly rejected others. There is a danger that this society, with its identity damaged by the Nazi past, may allow itself to become entangled in a deadly dance, when as a representative of law and order, it is inefficient in its caretaking function. If clear limits and values are not offered to these adolescents, they experience that which they have always experienced, and consequently their antisocial attitudes endure.

Summary

The violent environment of the extreme right offers male youths specific stability, which supports their adolescent self-system and at the same time intensifies personality malformations. Restructuring of the personality, development of a new we-feeling, coping with drive pressure, and ego syntonic reorganization of infantile conflicts are developmental challenges of adolescence. These overtax youths who have experienced continual trauma in their family and social environments. Histories of teenage skinheads show the processes of adaptation and assimilation which lead to establishing a grandiose self, a peer ideology, a self-reparative transformation of self-hatred into xenophobia, and a regressive sexual desire to lust for violence which mask the personality. With the deadly dance (a gang formation process) the developmental steps which lead to violence are described. A profile is presented to indicate some of the recurring features observed in the background and psychodynamics of skinheads in present-day Germany.

REFERENCES

Adorno, T. W. (1951), Die Freudsche Theorie und die Struktur faschistischen Propaganda (Freud's theories and the structure of fascist propaganda). *Psyche,* 24:486–508, 1970.

Blos, P. (1976), The split parental imago in adolescent social relations. *The Psychoanalytic Study of the Child,* 31:7–35. New Haven, CT: Yale University Press.

Chasseguet-Smirgel, I. (1975), *L'idéal de moi* (The Id ideal). Paris: Tchou.

Eissler, K. R. N. (1968), Weitere Bemerkungen zum Problem der KZ-Psychologie (Wide-ranging observations on the problem of KZ-Psychology). *Psyche,* 22:452–463.

Emde, R. N. (1984), Die endliche und die unendliche Entwicklung (Finite and infinite development). *Psyche,* 45:745–779.

Erdheim, M. (1984), *Die gesellschaftliche Produktion von Unbewußtheit* (The social creation of the unconscious). Frankfurt: Suhrkamp, 1991.

Fend, H. (1990), Vom Kind zum Jugendlichen (From child to youth). In: *Entwicklungspsychologie der Adoleszenz,* Vol. 1 (The evolution of adolescence). Stuttgart: Huber.

Gilmore, D. D. (1991), *Mythos Mann* (Mythical Man). München: Artemis und Winkler.

Giovacchini, P. (1978), The borderline aspects of adolescence and the borderline state. *Adol. Psychiatry,* 6:320–338.

Hacker, F. (1990), *Das Faschismus-Syndrom* (The fascist syndrome). Düsseldorf: Econ.

Hartmann, H. (1927), *Die Grundlagen der Psychoanalyse* (The foundations of psychoanalysis). Stuttgart: Klett, 1972.

Heitmeyer, W. (1987), *Rechtsextremistische Orientierungen bei Jugendlichen* (Right wing extremism amongst young people). Weinheim/München: Juventa.

——— (1988), Ökonomische soziale Alltagserfahrungen und rechtsextremistische Orientierungen bei Jugendlichen. In: *Risiko Jugend,* ed. F. Benseler, W. Heitmeyer, D. Pfeiffer, & D. Sengling. Münster: Votum, pp. 219–232.

——— (1992), *Rechtsextremistische Orientierungen bei Jugendlilchen* (Right-wing extremism amongst young people). Weinheim: Juventa.

Hochheimer, W. (1962–1963), Vorurteilsminderung in der Erziehung und die Prophylaxe des Antisemitismus (Reduction in prejudice in education and its prevention of Anti-Semitism). *Psyche,* 16:285–294.

Internationale Klassifikation psychischer Störungen (1993), *ICD-10, Kapitel V (F)* (World Health Organization). Bern: Huber.

Jacobson, E. (1964), *Das Selbst und die Welt der Objekte* (The self and the world of the object). Frankfurt: Suhrkamp, 1973.

Kernberg, O. F. (1975), *Borderlinestörungen und pathologischer Narzißmus* (Borderline disorder and pathological narcissism). Frankfurt: Suhrkamp, 1979.

Levi-Strauss, C. (1973), *Strukturale Anthropologie,* Vol. 2 (Structural Anthropology). Frankfurt: Suhrkamp, 1992.

Lowenfeld, H. (1937), Zur Psychologie des Faschismus (On the psychology of fascism). *Psyche,* 31:561–579, 1977.

Lowenfeld, Y. (1978), Eine Rettungsphantasie (A rescue fantasy). In: *Alexander Mitscherlich zu Ehren,* ed. S. Drews, R. Kluewer, A. Koehler-Weisker, M. Krueger-Zeul, K. Menne, & H. Vogel. Frankfurt: Suhrkamp, pp. 249–253.

Mitscherlich, A. (1970), Protest and revolution. *Psyche,* 24:510–520.

Mitscherlich-Nielsen, M. (1983), Antisemitismus, eine Männerkrankheit? (Antisemitism, mankind's illness?). *Psyche,* 37:41–54.

Morgenthaler, F. (1974), Die Stellung der Perversionen in Metapsychologie und Technik (The position of perversion in metapsychology and technique). *Psyche,* 8:1077–1098.

Müller-Braunschweig, H. (1985), Früher befiehl—zu Hitlers Wirkung im Deutschland der 30er Jahre (The former order—The effect of Hitler on Germany thirty years later). *Psyche,* 39:301–329.

Parin, P. (1978), Varum die Psychoanalytiker so ungern zu brennenden Zeitproblemen Stellung nehmen (Why is psychoanalysis so unwilling to confront the burning issue of the day?). *Psyche,* 32:301–399.

Piaget, J., & Inhelder, B. (1977), *Die Psychologie des Kindes* (The psychology of children). Frankfurt: Fischer.

Reimitz, M. (1989), Skinheads. In: *Zwischen Resignation und Gewalt* (Between renunciation and power), ed. M. Bock, M. Reimitz, H. E. Richter, W. Thiel, & H. J. Wirth. Opladen: Buderich Leske, pp. 183–186.

Sarnoff, C. F. (1987), *Psychotherapeutic Strategies in Late Latency through Early Adolescence.* Northvale, NJ: Jason Aronson.

Shatan, C. F. (1981), "Zivile" und "militärische" Realitätswahrnehmung ("Cruel" and "military" perception of reality). *Psyche,* 35:557–572.

——— (1983), Militarisierte Trauer und Rachezeremoniell (Militaristic mourning and ceremony of revenge). In: *Krieg und Frieden aus psychoanalytischer Sicht* (War and peace through psychoanalytic insight), ed. P. Passett & E. Modena. München: Piper, pp. 220–249.

Stein, H. F. (1990), The indispensable enemy and American-Soviet relations: In: *The Psychodynamics of International Relationships,* Vol. 1, ed. V. D. Volkan, D. A. Julius, & J. V. Montville. Toronto: Lexington Books, pp. 71–89.

Streeck-Fischer, A. (1992), Geil auf Gewalt: Adoleszenz und Rechtsextremismus (The luxury of might: Adolescence and right-wing extremism). *Psyche,* 46:745–768.

——— (1994a), "Wir sind die Kraft, die Deutschland sauber macht"—Oder eine Entstehung von Fremdenhaß und Gewalt als Gruppenporozeß ("We are the strength, Germany's authority" or the origins of hatred of outsiders and power in the group process). *Gruppenpsychother. Gruppendynamik,* 30:75–85.

——— (1994b), Männliche Adoleszenz, Fremdenhaß und seine selbstreparative Funktion am Beispiel jugendlicher rechtsextremer Skinheads (The male adolescent, hatred of outsiders, and his self-detachment function as an example of young right-wing extremist skinheads). *Praxis der Kinderpsychologie und Kinderpsychiatrie,* 43:259–266.

——— (1994c), Entwicklungslinien der Adoleszenz (Developmental antecedents of adolescence). *Psyche,* 48:509–528.

Wellmer, M. (1995), Fremdenfeindliche Einstellungen von Jugendlichen. Werkstattsbericht des Instituts für Sozialforschung und Lehrerbildung (Unknown enemies of young people's adjustment to workshop at the Institutes for Social Research and Education). Typescript.

Winnicott, D. W. (1965), *Reifungsprozesse und fördernde Umwelt* (The maturational processes and the facilitating environment). Frankfurt: Fischer, 1984.

Ziehe, T. (1975), *Pubertät und Narzißmus* (Puberty and narcissism). Frankfurt: EVA.

14
Adolescent
Survivors of the Holocaust

MAX SUGAR, M.D.

Although in the course of the twentieth century there have been many genocidal events—in Armenia, Iraq, China, Turkey, Greece, Spain, Bosnia, Mozambique, Nigeria, Russia, Rwanda, Burundi, Cambodia, and Nazi Germany—the best data available to date on genocide and its effects derive from the latter. In this chapter I will review the developmental effects on surviving adolescents who faced genocide in the ghettoes and concentration camps of the German Nazi regime. Since there is little direct focus on adolescents in the literature, the general remarks about camp survivors include adults and adolescents unless noted otherwise.

NORMATIVE ADOLESCENT DEVELOPMENT

As a background against which to reflect on the adolescent survivors' experiences, it may be useful to recall briefly some things about normative adolescence. In adolescence there are challenges and conflicts to be reworked and harmonized from previous developmental levels such as the preoedipal issues of dependency vs. autonomy; trust vs. mistrust; and the positive and

271

negative features from the oedipal stage. From latency there remain issues of developing industry versus inferiority, higher levels of object relations, beginning character formation, and superego development.

Normal adolescent mourning (Sugar, 1968) involves gradually giving up the infantile objects emotionally in a phasic process. In early adolescence there is the separation–protest phase with the simultaneous wish to separate and to restore or retain the infantile objects. This is often accompanied by angry, rebellious behavior. In the disorganization phase of midadolescence there is further distancing from the infantile objects and the adolescent's ego feels depleted. Then there are feelings of being worthless, empty, and inadequate. The adolescent may appear depressed, withdrawn or restless and often seeks new thrills or may be isolated. There may be resurgences of the wish to restore the tie with the infantile objects, but mostly there is recognition of the reality, and beginning acceptance of, the emotional shift away from, and decreasing dependency on, them. In late adolescence there is the reorganization phase with the wish for freedom from parents' and other authorities' restrictions; the need for exploring and managing reactions to the same and the opposite sex; the need to test one's omnipotentiality; and to arrive at a sense of fidelity and commitment to self and object choice.

Body image is reflected in self-image and identity, which make it a most significant part of adolescence. When chronic illness or other conditions interfere with the expectations of adolescence, it affects identity and body image (Sugar, 1990b).

For personality consolidation to occur in late adolescence, the youngster has to: (1) deal with residual trauma from childhood; (2) develop ego continuity; (3) establish one's sexual identity; and (4) resolve the second separation-individuation (Blos, 1974). These also mean taking responsibility for one's actions, and not attributing them to others. When character formation is evident by the end of adolescence, personality consolidation has occurred.

Concentration Camp Experiences
and Adolescent Development

Historically, the genocidal goal in a war has been the death of the target population which is perceived as the military enemy. The initial Nazi target was not a military force or a real enemy, but their own citizens who were helpless and defenseless whether educated or not; the mentally and physically handicapped, psychotics, and homosexuals, whether Jewish or not; and those not conforming to an idealized mythic fantasy of purity, such as the Jews and Gypsies. The specific goal of destroying the Jews and the Gypsies makes this behavior genocide, and not a war against the Jews or Gypsies. The term, *genocide*, which was first used during World War II, means destruction of a race or tribe (Mant, 1978). Later, the civilian Jewish and Gypsy populations of annexed or conquered countries became targets of genocide. The population of Poland and Russia were considered inferior, and if healthy, were placed in slave labor camps or concentration camps, as were Jews, Gypsies, and others who were strong enough to work until they died of exhaustion. The means the Nazis used can be considered as demoralization, destruction of identity, and then death. In some aspects this was similar to the genocide of the Cambodians by the Khmer Rouge from 1975 to 1979 when about 3 million of the 7 million Cambodians were exterminated. It involved debasement, especially of the urban and educated, and relocation to work in the countryside, followed by death.

In the medical literature there is no separation of Holocaust survivors into categories according to country of origin, length of exposure to degradation, or ghettoization prior to labor camp or concentration camp, length of incarceration, or individual experiences. Marrus (1985) details a varied pattern of genocidal effort and effect according to the occupied country, its leader's cooperation or resistance to the Nazis, and the presence of a population that supported the Nazis' genocidal plan or resisted it and assisted the Jews. Since the Nazis were concerned about the effect on the German population of knowing about the destruction of their own citizens, it was done secretly and most of the extermination camps were in Poland.

Of Germany's pre-World War II population of 500,000 Jews, 300,000 escaped extermination primarily by emigration in 1933 and 1938. Western Greece was initially occupied by the Italian army and its Jews were not deported due to Italian protection, while the Bulgarians occupying Thrace and part of Macedonia did little to aid the German's Final Plan until Spring 1943. When the Germans replaced the Italian troops after the latter had rebelled against the fascists, and hanged Mussolini, and joined the Allies, the Jews of the western area of Greece were deported to Auschwitz with the loss of most of the 80,000 Jews of Greece (Stavroulakis and DeVinney, 1992). A similar situation occurred in Italy and in Hungary.

In Poland, where the Jews had no general support from the local population and the country was governed by the Nazis for nearly six years, almost all 3 million of its Jews were annihilated along with 2 million Poles. About 2 million Russians and Russian POWs were also murdered in the camps. Of the 6 million Jews in the camps, only 100,000 survived, and of these, 4,000 were children (Friedman, 1949). Matussek (1975, pp. 18–20) details significant differences among the concentration camps in severity of conditions and the variety of arrangements for harshness to and annihilation of victims.

STAGES OF REACTION
IN THE CONCENTRATION CAMPS

Before being imprisoned there were years of degradation, assaults, restrictions, and threats to life to the Jews. Incarceration was frightening and perplexing to all since no crime had been committed, while terror and deception were used to get the victims' maximum cooperation.

The victims usually came into the extermination camps (Auschwitz, Birkenau, Belcec, Treblinka, Majdanek, Sobibor, etc.) from the ghettoes, or exhausted from work in slave labor camps. On arrival in the Nazi concentration camps, those younger than 14, pregnant, physically handicapped, chronically ill, or over 50 were put to death immediately (Cohen, 1953).

Adolescents and adults who were strong and able to work were kept alive for a time for that purpose and often sent to slave labor camps, or taken directly from the platform at the extermination camps and put to work there immediately. Work in the munitions or chemical plants was for the Nazi war machine and posed an ethical dilemma, while other work was meaningless and repetitious.

Cohen (1953) described the stages of camp life as follows: if the facts of the camp's goal were known beforehand, there was an initial phase of "I don't belong," with acute depersonalization; then came death anxiety which was followed by apathy for several weeks. This was followed by a short euphoric mood, after which there was a depression lasting for three to six months (Cohen, 1953). There were thousands who died of emotional and physical exhaustion in the early stage of incarceration (i.e., giving up due to loss of family or simply being overwhelmed with the horror of their situation) (Des Pres, 1976). The suicides in the Nazi camps (labor and concentration) and after liberation were poorly reported (Ryn, 1986) although there were many.

DAILY ROUTINES
IN NAZI CONCENTRATION CAMPS

There was no change of clothes and personal hygiene was limited by the Nazis. Sleep was restricted to about four hours. Individuality and identity were erased by having all body and head hair shaved on entrance to the camp; all personal items were removed; tattooed numbers were used for identification instead of names;

and no privacy existed even in bathing or at the latrine. The future, hope of a future, and a sense of time were denied the persecuted by the absence of clocks and calendars, or explanations for the persecution. They soon learned that survival in the labor camps was based on working and being healthy enough to continue to do so for fourteen to eighteen hours per day (Cohen, 1953; De Pres, 1976). This led to daily inspection of themselves and requests for confirmation of health by fellow prisoners (Levi, 1969).

In the killing camps there was only a short interlude before extermination. Auschwitz had signs clearly indicating that the only way out was through the chimneys, and that the stay for Jews was three weeks. Denial was a major defense since it dulled awareness and decreased panic attacks.

Des Pres (1976) detailed the sadistic means by which the SS guards and criminal kapos sought to attain complete degradation of the victims. One approach was to provide only two latrines for 30,000 victims to use on schedule only, twice a day without any toilet paper. The latrines were open ditches twelve feet deep without seats and with only a railing to hold onto while performing excretory functions in full view of the guards and the opposite sex. Punishment ensued if attempts were made to relieve themselves at any other time, or if they used their soup bowls for this during the night. This routine was not altered by the epidemics of typhus or dysentery. The victims were caked with their own excrement and its odor was constantly with them.

Guards toyed with the victims by making them urinate over groups of others who were supine, or forcing victims to urinate into the mouths of others. Another game was to stop a prisoner on his way to the latrine, force him to squat to do deep knee-bends until he "exploded," beat him, then allow him to use the latrine. When prisoners were at the latrine the kapos often pushed them into it, which led to suffocation. Among the incarcerated who cleaned these pits at night, some fell in nightly (about ten per night in one camp). But helping them was forbidden, and the corpses were not extricated until the next morning. Des Pres (1976) indicates that the goal was loss of the prisoners' morale in order to deter the development of feeling for, or cooperation with, others. Those who washed themselves and maintained a sense of dignity in spite of all had a better chance of survival. When this ceased, it was symptomatic and predictive of death (Des Pres, 1976, pp. 57–64).

Adaptation to camp routine was difficult since the SS guards changed their rules capriciously, and invited spying and betrayal among prisoners. The condition of Jewish victims was the worst since they were routinely degraded more than others by the SS guards, and they often witnessed, or expected, the murder of family members in the same or other camps (Cohen, 1953). The Polish Jews were treated worse than the German Jews (Matussek, 1975, p. 26). Decreased memory occurred after a while (Bettelheim, 1943). A ray of hope was helpful to survival and might come in the form of a kindness from another victim (Davidson, 1979), or work on an intellectual task (Bettelheim, 1943), or revengeful fantasies (Frankl, 1959), or luck (Matussek, 1975, p. 32; Davidson, 1979).

It was well known that to be ill in the camps was very risky since often there was little chance of recovery, and afterward, selection was for extermination, not for work (Cohen, 1953). However, there were many with illnesses, and those under 20 had more "psychological syndromes." The disorders of adults and adolescents are listed in Table 14.1 according to Matussek (1975, p. 61) which Des Pres (1976) confirms.

Many medical experiments were made on the prisoners such as exposure to typhus, malaria, freezing, high altitude conditions, mustard gas, phosgene gas, seawater, and sulfas; futile operations were done to see whether bone, muscle, or nerves would regenerate; there was bone transplantation, sterilization, and euthanasia of mental patients (Des Pres, 1976).

Calorie intake varied by location. In one camp it was 1300 to 1400 calories/day, while at Dachau it was 1017 calories daily in September 1944, and 533 calories in April 1945 (Cohen, 1953). In 1939 at Dachau the prisoners were given 1800 calories per day for work which required 3300 calories for the 12- to 18-hour work days (Bettelheim, 1943).

TABLE 14.1
Physical and Mental Disorders While Incarcerated

	%
Head Injuries from Maltreatment	48
Epidemics	28
Chest Disorders	26
Cardiac Disorders	29
Rheumatic Complaints	26
Dyspeptic Symptoms	26
Signs of Hunger Dystrophy (cachexia, polyuria edema)	29
Bacterial Infections	21
Injuries from Maltreatment	21
Spinal Column Symptoms	10
Infections	7
Brief Febrile Infection	10
Frostbite (feet)	2
Permanent Anxiety State	28
Depressive Moods	31
Suicidal Thoughts	8

Source: P. Matussek, *Internment in Concentration Camps and Its Consequences*, New York: Springer-Verlag, 1975, p. 61, modified. Reprinted by permission.

With an unbalanced, very low calorie diet during the first year of incarceration by the Nazis, along with extreme physical exertion for 14 or more hours daily, and finally an unbalanced diet of 800 or fewer calories a day for those who survived through the last year of the war (Matussek, 1975), it is not surprising that there was emaciation. This aided apathy (numbing), and death by starvation followed for many. The finding that oral needs were primary for those who survived is readily understandable.

According to Matussek (1975, p. 30, citing Cayrol, 1959) women (age not specified) were more affected and stressed than men. However, Carmil and Carel (1986) and Nadler and Ben-Shushan (1989) found that 40 years later male survivors were worse off psychologically than females. Danieli (1982) explained this on the basis of the experience of being helpless in the concentration camp which is contrary to the male's image of being a strong protector and provider.

The victims experienced a loss of sexual interest and impotence. Sexual jokes were absent and replaced by scatological ones. All the women had amenorrhea. Frankl (1959) and Cohen (1953)

reported no heterosexual activity in the concentration camps between the incarcerated. Dream content was not erotic but of hunger and food. Masturbation and homosexuality were widespread,
the latter especially among the SS guards and kapos (Cayrol,
1959, cited in Matussek, 1975). The camps had brothels that the
SS guards and kapos used. According to Cayrol (1959, cited in
Matussek, 1975) the prostitutes were professionals, but Cohen
(1953) states that the brothels had no true prostitutes, just coerced prisoners. The prisoners rarely went there, and those who
did wanted to just talk to a woman, since the men and women
were segregated. Survival was the main issue that preoccupied
the victims.

The camp population was unstable since those working today
might be tomorrow's corpses in the gas chambers, or relocated
to other (labor) camps. Family members were separated, and if
together, it was briefly since the elderly were often executed in
the presence of relatives or taken to the gas chambers immediately. Being left to one's own devices might mean suicide (De
Pres, 1976; Davidson, 1985; Ryn, 1986).

In order to survive, youngsters moved quickly from whatever
stage of latency or adolescence they were in at the onset of the
Holocaust into premature pseudoadulthood during the ghetto
stage. However, a few adolescent features were evident. Some
formed groupings of two or three as adolescents usually do (Davidson, 1979). Some of them became the leaders who initiated,
or continued, resistance, or escaped to become partisan fighters,
or attempted escapes and revolts in the labor and concentration
camps. There were escapes and uprisings such as in the Warsaw
ghetto, and the camps at Auschwitz and Buchenwald. The prisoners also burned down the camps at Treblinka and Sobibor, and
blew up one of the crematoria at Auschwitz. But freedom was
short-lived for most, and few escaped for long (Des Pres, 1976).

THE NEED TO BEAR WITNESS

The Germans' fear of discovery led them to begin opening the
mass graves and burning the bodies at Treblinka. Had this been

achieved, there would have been no record of Treblinka's horrors, or that it even existed. But the Sonderkommandos, made up of the persecuted, organized a revolt in Treblinka and burned down the camp on August 2, 1943, with the goal of memorializing Treblinka and the events therein. Forty survived and bore witness to their experiences, which was a compulsion among some survivors (Des Pres, 1976, p. 38).

Lifton (1972, p. 519) has called the need to bear witness, "the anxiety of responsibility." Des Pres (1976) lists many who wrote under intense pressure to bear witness. Levi (1969, p. 36) described his almost fatal indifference to survival until another victim told him that "even in this place we can survive, and therefore we must want to survive to tell the story, to bear witness."

SURVIVAL AND LUCK

Many survivors mention luck as a major factor in their survival. Sometimes altruism and luck combined as happened on one occasion in Buchenwald. When a transport arrived from Hungary with 410 boys, the resistance leaders in the camp bargained with the SS and convinced them that if these youngsters were allowed to live they would be excellent workers. Luckily the SS was agreeable. Each youngster then had a designated underground member to provide food, clothing, and caring. This resulted in each of these children being alive at liberation (Des Pres, 1976, p. 128).

CASE PRESENTATION

A 15-year-old was beaten and insulted routinely by his civilian German overseer in a labor camp making munitions until he could no longer tolerate the abuse. When it occurred next he struck and injured the man with a handy piece of equipment. Was this suicidal? Perhaps, since he knew it meant immediate death by hanging. However, he denied it and felt he was safe by threatening to inform the camp commandant of the corruption which was rife among the camp guards and supervisors.

When this threat failed, a German woman, a junior supervisor, whom he did not know, interceded to claim that he was "her Jew." Since he belonged to her they could not damage her property. Apparently, at some risk to herself she saved his life by putting him in her protective custody to work with her in the kitchen.

To the extent that the high-risk youngsters in the study by Werner and Smith (1982) were "able to elicit predominantly positive responses from the environment, they were found to be stress-resistant at each stage of their life cycle." Perhaps the youngster in this case had this ability, which influenced the German woman to save him. For this youngster luck may have also been a factor.

FORCED MARCHES

With the advance of the Russian army westward, the Nazis treated prisoners they could not leave behind as hostages. The SS forced them to march in the winter of 1944–1945 from camps in Poland into Czechoslovakia and Germany. These became death marches during which a great many of the persecuted died of starvation or were shot for falling behind. For example, of the 60,000 prisoners who left Auschwitz, about a third arrived in the next camp in Czechoslovakia (Cohen, 1953).

AFTER LIBERATION

For some, liberation meant revenge, and some killed their guards immediately, as did U.S. troops on liberating Dachau (Beuchner, 1986). For others, it meant death since they were unsupervised initially in their food intake by the liberating troops, gorged themselves, and died. Others suicided (Ryn, 1986).

After liberation there was the ultimate debacle when the survivors learned that their hoped for reunion with family members was a fantasy since they had been exterminated, and their town of origin no longer knew, cared for, or wanted them. Although

displaced persons (DP) camps were provided, societal indifference, avoidance, and denial of their experiences prevailed in Europe (Danieli, 1982).

Des Pres (1976, p. 116) challenges Bettelheim's (1943) observations that identification with the aggressor occurred among the
survivors. The reliability of Bettelheim's statements has come under more critical scrutiny recently, and raises the question of the
veracity of his pronouncements (Pollak, 1997).

After liberation the survivors now also had to contend with
shame and guilt about their camp experiences, pent-up rage
about their loss of liberty, losses (of family and personal possessions), humiliation, and helplessness. The adolescents displaced
this in various hostile and negative attitudes and behavior to their
helpers, protectors, and therapists for a number of years after
liberation (Klein, 1973; Sterba, 1968).

Many who left the DP camps for Palestine in 1946 and 1947
were prevented from entering it by the British who interned them
on Cyprus. The survivors now had a repetition of the trauma of
the Nazi concentration camps. Among these adolescents (up to
age 18) Friedman (1949) found a few cases of psychosis, many
reactive depressions, conversion reactions, and hypochondriacal
symptoms. Fifty to 60 percent of the adolescents requesting medical treatment had psychosomatic symptoms. These youngsters
showed fatigue; loss of sexuality (which they had regained after
liberation), including masturbation; inability to cry; excessive
sleepiness (lasting for days); detachment; and shallow emotions.

Most survivors spent two to four years in the DP camps, had
many moves and had to learn new languages and work skills.
My conjecture is that after liberation their sense of identity was
probably still fragile, along with fears of recurrent atrocities,
numbing, reexperiencing, memory difficulty, concentration
problems, sleep disturbances, startle reactions, guilt, suspicious-
ness, and intensification of symptoms, as in PTSD. A small percent
became psychotic. There is no doubt that many had serious physical problems.

The youngsters under 20 had more difficulty in deciding on,
or training for, an occupation, and had more job insecurity than

the older survivors. The young who were successful in work took a job just to be active, threw themselves compulsively into the job, and changed jobs often (Matussek, 1975, p. 156). This appears to have been a hypomanic defense against their depression, as well as the wish to make up for their lost years.

ADOLESCENT MOURNING

The adolescent Holocaust survivors had the additional complication of being unable to mourn their losses, especially of parents. With the family destroyed they could not proceed through normal adolescent mourning and the development of gradual emotional separation-individuation from parents (Blos, 1962; Sugar, 1968). They could not mourn the actual dead since cathartic rituals were prohibited in the concentration camps, and there were only unknown or mass graves. If they had manifested appropriate horror, rage, and grief at executions while in the camps, it would have endangered their own lives (Grubrich-Simitis, 1979).

Not infrequently following a parent's death, the adolescent has an academic decline, misconduct in school, steals, or is truant. Normal adolescent mourning (Sugar, 1968) (or a trial mourning) for the infantile objects, that is, the gradual decathexis of the image of the parents, is a prerequisite for the later ability to mourn, since one has then learned how to give up a major love object (Wolfenstein, 1966).

The loss of parents in adolescence may lead to an absence of mourning, covert denial of the reality of loss (Fleming and Altschul, 1963) and continued fantasies of finding the lost parents (Jacobson, 1965). These defense mechanisms avoid the painful process of decathexis of the lost parent, and instead there develops an intensified cathexis of the parent (Wolfenstein, 1966) with overidealization. The youngster does not cry, and there is an interference with the expression of affect, with isolation of affect from thoughts. In addition, the usual, previous adolescent ambivalence to the parent (now departed) is split off, with the hostile feelings directed to others in the environment, bringing about alienation (Sterba, 1968; Klein, 1973).

Since there was no opportunity for a continued relationship with a parent-surrogate in the concentration camps, the adolescent was without the emotional support to help him or her through this and be able to continue adolescent development. From this it appears that a developmental arrest occurred at the stage in which the adolescent was at the time of their parents' deaths. This indicates the need for the continuing relationship with the parent in order for the adolescent's development to go forward.

The adolescents in the concentration camp thus had an interference with normal adolescent mourning due to forced separation from parents, daily fear of death, and the horrors; and if the parents themselves were dead they could not mourn them internally or externally. If they were uncertain about the parents' fate the youngsters were still held in the limbo of the stage of adolescent development they were in at the onset of incarceration by being unable to decathex the parents in the normal fashion and move forward to new objects. Later, there was the repetition of increased dependency for those youngsters whose hopes for reunion with family members were shattered after liberation when they were placed in DP camps.

The youngsters who were in concentration camps between ages 12 and 20, and were seen after liberation by Sterba (1968), were very dissatisfied and negative about everything, including the food, and the younger ones could not establish a good relationship with a foster parent or relatives. They felt unwanted and excluded, and acted out aggressively, even when their wish was granted to move to another foster home or to a relative. They had separation problems and disclosed information with difficulty. Many had somatic symptoms and depression. She felt their neurotic symptoms were reactions to their concentration camp experiences where they had to control themselves at all costs to survive. But in their new situation where they felt safe, they expressed their anger and wished for immediate gratification

(Sterba, 1968). This seems to have been rage about their losses which was now able to be expressed in a safe place.

ADOLESCENT DEVELOPMENT
IN SURVIVORS OF CONCENTRATION CAMPS

By comparing the late adolescence of those working or in college in the United States with those in Nazi ghettoes or concentration camps, the severity of the developmental limitation of the latter two groups may be seen in Table 14.2. "The ghetto robbed me of my youth" said one 16-year-old girl after liberation (Matussek, 1975, p. 27).

For some there was another opportunity for further development. A group of adolescent females who, through luck, were

TABLE 14.2
Late Adolescence Compared

| | In United States | | In Nazi | |
	Working	College	Ghetto	Conc. Camp
Dependency	↓[a]	↑[b]	↑	↑
Learning Opportunity	↓	↑	↓	↓
Capacity for Self-Observation	↓	↑	↓	↓
Consolidation of Character	↑	↓	↑	↑
Sense of Independence	↑	↓	↓	↓
Autonomy	↑	↓	↓	↓
Opportunity for Identification with Mentors	↓	↑	↓	↓
Try Out Different Ego Ideals	↓	↑	↓	↓
Completion of Sense of Identity	↑	↓	↓	↓

[a] ↓ = decreased
[b] ↑ = increased

together for a number of months in Auschwitz, developed groups of five with "intense mutual aid and protectiveness which continued during their next $1^1/_2$ years in a slave labor camp until their liberation" (Davidson, 1979, p. 400). This also involved large-group supportive behavior. Male adolescents formed two- to three-person friendships in the camps which aided their survival. They helped each other steal food, shared everything, and joined large groups when required (Davidson, 1979).

As adolescents, their need for, and use of, peer group interaction was age-appropriate and supported them through the horrors of the concentration camp. The dangers seemed to be a challenge and competition for them, especially the males (Davidson, 1979). For those adolescent survivors who were kept in special group homes in England (boys) and Czechoslovakia (girls) for a number of months and then supported for several years after in England (Davidson, 1979; Gilbert, 1996), some may have had further adolescent development, though delayed. Most of these have been closely involved with one another ever since, and have done well with relationships, vocations, and family life (Solkoff, 1992; Gilbert, 1996).

Although I found no mention in the literature of body image concerns by these adolescents, it seems unlikely that the youngsters were not troubled about deterioration of their bodies with emaciation, illness, and absent sexual function (Sugar, 1990b). Levi's (1969) point about daily inspection of themselves does not specify whether it was about adults only, but it would seem reasonable to consider that adolescents were also involved in this.

In the concentration camps these youngsters faced genocide and had no certainty that they still had families from whom to separate and individuate. Whatever ego ideals existed were present from latency years or early adolescence before incarceration, just as whatever ego, superego, adaptive skills and beginning character traits they had were residua from parental tutelage.

Table 14.3 provides a view of the possibility of completing the tasks of late adolescence in concentration camps.

Considering all these features, was it possible for these youngsters to have an adolescence? I should think not. Their adolescence was foreshortened and arrested. The luxury of being

TABLE 14.3
Completion of Tasks of Late Adolescence
in Concentration Camp Survivors

Tasks of Late Adolescence	Concentration Camp Prisoners
Consolidation	No
Separating from Parents	Yes
Identity Formation	No
Achieving Genital Primacy	No
Sexual Identity	No
Development of a Time Perspective	No
Commitment to a Life Goal	No
Development of Intimacy	No
Development of Friendships	Yes
Development of Harmonizing of Ego, Superego, and Ego Ideal	No

dependent, rebelling, changing ego ideals, and experimentation was not available. They became pseudoadults and endured massive repeated terror, humiliation, and atrocities, with threats to their identity and lives for years.

It seems that those adolescents with murdered parents, massive repeated trauma, and without parent surrogates had a developmental arrest. This was due to the massive trauma and equally to the absence of normative adolescent mourning (Sugar, 1968) and the second separation–individuation stage (Blos, 1962, pp. 132–136). Bearing in mind their displaced hostility to and distrust of helpers and therapists, this view leads to the consideration that this behavior was a defense against retraumatization (i.e., object loss). Their attitude and behavior could also be considered as signs of hope (Winnicott, 1957) since they felt enough trust to express anger now about their losses to those closest and most helpful to them. With this displacement, some may have been able to resume their adolescent development with rebellious, ambivalent, and hostile attitudes and behavior to their helpers, parent substitutes, who accepted it. This probably led to a different and delayed, but something akin to, adolescence for them. With this, I would submit that normative adolescent development and consolidation cannot occur without the presence of parents or parent surrogates.

TRANSFER TO THE NEXT GENERATION

A review of the literature of the effect on the children of survivors of the Holocaust is inconclusive. According to some authors (Rakoff, Sigal, and Epstein, 1967; Klein, 1973; Davidson, 1980; Ryn, 1990) the adolescent concentration camp survivors had their massive trauma in adolescence, and many had difficulty when their own children entered adolescence, whether Jewish or not. Many of their adolescents had problems such as depression, personality disturbances, alcoholism, and suicide. These parents were depressed, preoccupied with their trauma, lacked the ability to control or relate to the youngsters, and were overprotective. Often they overvalued their adolescents as representative of the lost relatives. The parents overestimated their children's abilities and encouraged them to do what they had been unable to do in their own adolescence. They had bilateral separation problems.

Dasberg (1987) summarized studies which show that the traumatic family milieu created by mourning and demanding parents affected the offspring. He noted that the extent of parental trauma correlated with that in offspring; the youngsters lacked psychosocial maturity. Survivors felt their children had to be high achievers to compensate for the parental losses.

Although these reports point to a specific relationship between the pathology of the adolescent offspring of survivors and the massive trauma of the survivors, most of the reports have no control groups, such as adolescents from other immigrant groups, and usually the adolescents are not separated by gender. Where studies have included a control group it seems that "the effect of immigrant status is as important as Holocaust experience in determining differences in psychological adjustment in offspring" (Solkoff, 1992, p. 356). The absence of a transmission

effect in the study by Major (1996) that compared second generation Norwegian Jews with a control group corroborates this assessment.

However, the analysis of some adolescent offspring of Holocaust survivors has illuminated facets of their development and
ego functions that are of particular interest. Grubrich-Simitis
(1984) noted that the permeability of their ego boundaries in
areas related to trauma endured by either one or both parents
probably serves as a defense; and that they have an impaired
ability to use metaphor. These were subject to positive alteration
with analysis.

COUNTERTRANSFERENCE

Many physicians minimized the survivors' emotional problems
and considered them as organic or preexisting. Later they viewed
their symptoms as a "psycho-organic condition" due to the Holocaust experience. This had a number of stages, but ultimately
revealed its organic nature as dementia, or in characterological
features such as encephalopathy, epilepsy, and organic psychoses
(Ryn, 1990). Survivors were diagnosed as presenile dementia
(Thygesen, 1980), refugee neurosis (Pedersen, 1948), repatria-
tion neurosis (Eitinger, 1961), pension neurosis, and dependency
neurosis. Compensation was disallowed for these, but presenile
dementia and other physical diagnoses qualified for pensions by
the German government (Matussek, 1975). The guidelines of the
West German government for compensation allowed only a maximum of 35 percent disability for psychiatric diagnoses.

In the evaluations of those seeking pensions, by general prac-
titioners and specialists for the West German Compensation
Board after the war, psychiatrists in many different countries gave
the fewest diagnoses and the lowest rates of pension awards, as
Table 14.4 shows (Matussek, 1975).

TABLE 14.4

Case Rates of 60 Percent Awards for Disability
in Victims by Physicians' Group

	%
General Practitioners	>50
Public Health M.D.	>32
Internists	27
Psychiatrists	9.6

Source: P. Matussek, *Internment in Concentration Camps and Its Consequences,* New York: Springer-Verlag, 1975, pp. 75–76, modified. Reprinted by permission.

Matussek (1975, p. 86) lists eight diagnoses given by twelve physicians to concentration camp patients after liberation, such as asthenia, concentration camp syndrome, survivor syndrome (Niederland, 1968), and organic brain syndrome. Matussek (1975) notes the obvious and usual pattern as if it represents pathology when he states that women reintegrated socially through early marriage, more frequently than men, who reintegrated socially through work. A number of reports (Klein, Zellermayer, and Shanan, 1963; Trautman, 1971) remark on the survivors' early marriages to unsuitable people whom they hardly knew, since they had often just met in the DP camps after liberation. Trautman (1971) views this as premature behavior in an effort to reestablish a family or as an expression of sexuality. These remarks seem paternalistic, prejudiced, and indicative of a negative countertransference. But Matussek (1975) disagrees with these authors to note that these marriages were not correlated with marital disharmony and had only a 6 to 8 percent divorce rate (Matussek, 1975, p. 181; Kahana, Harel, and Kahana, 1988).

Bettelheim (1943), Cohen (1953), and Niederland (1968) consider that there was regression, loss, or silence of the superego, loss of compassion, and loss of caring about others among the persecuted. To consider that all the concentration camp victims regressed (as if psychotic) may be pejorative and reflects the authors' countertransference problems. Des Pres (1976, p. 31) provides details which support this view, and disagrees with

Bettelheim (1943), Cohen (1953), and Niederland (1968). He indicates refinement of conscience, return to God, victim groups helping each other (even on the death marches) with kindness, food, medicines, messages, and stealing ammunition and weapons for uprisings at the risk of their own lives.

CASE ILLUSTRATION

In one case a patient stated that as an adolescent on the death march from Auschwitz he gave up and lay down in the snow to die. However, another adolescent whom he had befriended and helped in the camp, pulled him up, and dragged him along, reassuring him all the while. They both made it to freedom and are still friends.

In addition, a strong "gift morality" and "bread morality" were present (Des Pres, 1976, pp. 140–142). Those who did not come into groups failed to survive the routine of daily life. Matussek (1975, pp. 36, 37) supports the fact that friendships existed. The need to help one another seemed as fundamental to survival as the need for help, according to De Pres (1976). The groups united, though with great caution and difficulty to "organize," that is, disobey the Germans (De Pres, 1976, pp. 104–106) and help each other, which was against the rules (pp. 67–147).

In psychiatric reports on combat infantry, I have not seen statements about regression, or sexual activity during combat. The incontinence that infantrymen often have in combat does not signify regression but is rather a reaction of the autonomic nervous system to fear.

Perhaps there were various levels of regression among the survivors so that although regression occurred (in those who became psychotic, or gave up and became "musselmen"), for the majority of survivors there was no primary process thinking, or return to a previous stage of development or function due to intrapsychic issues. Had there been universal regression, then uprisings, the burning of a camp, and the blowing up of a crematorium could not have occurred; nor could there have been a "gift" or "bread" morality in which people shared their resources. Only those survivors who required therapy or sought pensions from the West German government were evaluated psychiatrically.

For the victims there was a forced dependency with abandonment of much socialization and acculturation at the point of a gun. It seems that just as the combat infantryman adapts to conditions in order to fight and survive, so, too, did the concentration camp victims. Just as the artist uses regression in the service of the ego (Kris, 1944) to be able to create, here, too, the victims' regression was in the service of creativity for survival—the ego's major function. They did this by using their limited options to cope with capricious, terrorizing, sadistic captors in a living hell. Their coping efforts do not appear as a sign of neurosis or psychosis, but of adaptation to the worst of extreme conditions. However, the experiences may have affected their character development (Carmil and Carel, 1986; Nadler and Ben-Shushan, 1989).

In the study by Leon, Butcher, Kleinman, Goldberg, and Almagor (1981), survivor guilt was not apparent, in contrast to the statement by Krystal and Niederland (1968) that it was present in 92 percent of their patients. Niederland's (1968) remarks about survivor guilt as unresolved grief and mourning support Wolfenstein's (1966) and mine (see above). However, Niederland (1968) adds that beneath these feelings of guilt were "repressed rage and resentment against the lost parents for failing to protect" them (p. 314). This appears to point to the survivor's feeling of helplessness, which was paramount. While I agree that there was some survivor guilt, a part of that covered up the feeling of helplessness. Since the feeling of helplessness, which is related to infantile states, is much more painful and threatening to self-esteem and identity, the ego represses and denies this with guilt feelings. Then the phrase survivor guilt supplants it. In an effort to help these patients with their sense of helplessness, the therapist risks countertransference difficulties due to experiencing their very painful feelings of helplessness in trial identification (Sugar, 1988).

The liberation troops were initially appalled by, and contemptuous of, the walking skeletal survivors of the concentration camps. This was followed by guilt, compassion, and efforts to help (Prescott, 1986; *Times-Picayune*, 1995). There is also a tendency in the therapist to despise the sufferer, as if to distance oneself from hearing about others dehumanizing people (Eissler, 1967); to avoid learning that we, as therapists, fear losing contact with our good internal objects (Grubrich-Simitis, 1981); to avoid the intense feelings of helplessness aroused, and the question "What would I have done there?" (Sugar, 1988). The countertransference issues also include denial, avoidance, revulsion, projection, and rejection (Hoppe, 1967).

There is also the possibility of equal but opposite interfering countertransference reactions consisting of overprotectiveness, overdoing, and avoiding. This may be in the areas of confrontation or interpretation since it may be unpleasant to treat these patients. The therapist also has the personal task of surviving and not succumbing to the survival anxiety of the patient (Winnicott, 1957).

THE SURVIVOR'S DIAGNOSIS

The Nazis' behavior to the Holocaust victims was so inhuman that there are no comparisons, although Japanese treatment of the people in countries they conquered, and of Allied POWs in World War II are similar. The Germans mistreated POWs in the Allied forces, especially Jews and Russians, whom they removed to extermination camps. But other POWs were better treated than those of the Japanese, among whom there was a higher morbidity and mortality rate. The POWs in both German and Japanese POW camps had a higher frequency of PTSD than the non-POW combat soldiers. However, PTSD could not be forecast based on family history of mental illness, having had adjustment problems, or severe childhood trauma (Speed, Engdahl, Schwartz, and Eberly, 1989). However, torture, beatings, and weight loss as a POW were the best predictors of PTSD in World War II American POWs

(Speed et al., 1989) and their symptoms and diagnoses persist 50 years later. These conditions, and worse, were the daily lot of the concentration camp victims.

Forty years after the Holocaust, adolescent survivors had suspicion, and compared to controls, lower scores on emotional stability, self-discipline, self-control, spontaneous emotional expression, energy level, openness to change, dominance, and assertiveness (Nadler and Ben-Shushan, 1989). They also had a slightly higher degree of emotional disturbance than nonpatient survivors (Carmil and Carel, 1986). It seems to me that these are not specific to camp survivors, but are part of PTSD in reaction to the repeated experience of persecution, witnessing killings, and death threats.

When Kuch and Cox (1992) examined Holocaust survivors at age 62 (mean), some of whom were adolescents at the onset of persecution, they found that 46 percent of the cohort had PTSD 43 years later. The survivors had had minimal psychiatric care, but more than half were on minimal doses of benzodiazepines. Yehuda, Kahana, Southwick, and Giller (1994) reported that nonpatient adult Holocaust survivors with PTSD scored higher on depressive scales than those without PTSD. Their character structure was altered by the mind-numbing experiences according to Koenig (1964), Nadler and Ben-Shushan (1989), Krell (1990), Ryn (1990), and Robins, Rapport-Bar-Sever, and Rapport (1994). This is similar to American POWs and combat veterans with PTSD (Southwick, Yehuda, and Giller, 1993).

Posttraumatic stress disorder, somatic symptoms, and negative affect were noted in former U.S. POWs 20 to 40 years posttrauma (Engdahl, Harkness, Eberly, Page, and Brelinski, 1993). Among former U.S. POWs 35 years later, cognitive deficits, somatic symptoms, suspicion, confusion, isolation, detachment, and hostility were found (Sutker, Winstead, Galina, and Allain, 1991). Bremner, Scott, Delaney, Southwick, Mason, Johnson, Innis, McCarthy, and Charney (1993) observed deficits in short-term memory among Vietnam veterans with PTSD.

The diagnosis of PTSD has not been used as the primary one for the Holocaust survivors in the literature I have reviewed, but as an additional one (Kuch and Cox, 1992; Yehuda et al., 1994).

Essentially the Jews had been POWs since Germany began war on them in 1933, along with the Poles (since 1939), and the Russian POWs (since 1941), until 1945. I suggest that due to the catastrophic conditions endured, probably a majority of them developed PTSD.

Thus, it appears that adolescent survivors of the Holocaust have much in common with U.S. survivors of combat, and more so with those who were in Japanese POW camps. This is not intended to equate Japanese POW camps with, or minimize the horrors visited on, the Nazi concentration camp victims, but to bring the psychiatric condition into the fold. Posttraumatic stress disorder may occur with varying degrees of severity and comorbidity just as with any other condition. Not all survivors of the concentration camps had all the same experiences or the same exact outcome. Nevertheless, "Their youth is shattered by the trauma, and their old age is overshadowed by its aftereffects" (Nadler and Ben-Shushan, 1989).

The survivors developed symptoms in the concentration camps (Table 14.1), and after liberation further symptoms developed, often hypochondriacal. These symptoms all fit in the category of POWs with PTSD, with or without major depression or psychosis (DSM-IV, APA, 1994).

In treating such patients, the therapist needs to attempt gradual clarification of the actual events, including questions and confrontation. In other words, it is important for the dyad to accept the concentration camp experience as authentic. This means the therapist has to resist the need to avoid the anticipated, and actual, pain and anxiety induced by hearing about the real events. Otherwise, trial identifications with the patient and empathy are withheld and a "conspiracy of silence" develops (Krystal and Niederland, 1968).

Considering the various countertransference difficulties in evaluating or treating these patients empathetically (Grubrich-Simitis, 1981) in the early postliberation years, it seems that these issues still operate just as intensely today in all who enter this territory.

Viewing the survivors' conditions per DSM-IV in the same category as POWs with PTSD, and major depression, etc., as due to the extreme trauma to which they were subjected, provides the foundation for the first principle for their therapy. This consists of linking the symptoms with the events, and explaining them as a normal reaction to a most abnormal situation. This approach would relieve fears of being tainted, crazy, having a bad childhood or bad parents, or needing an organic diagnosis to obtain compensation.

Based on her experience, Grubrich-Simitis (1984) was optimistic about the therapeutic effect of psychoanalytic treatment of adolescent Holocaust survivors. In a research endeavor, Pennebaker, Barger, and Tiebout (1989) found that the Holocaust survivors who revealed their severe traumas were healthier in the following year than those who withheld such material.

REFERENCES

American Psychiatric Association (1994), *Diagnostic and Statistical Manual,* 4th (DSM-IV). Washington, DC: American Psychiatric Press.

Bettelheim, B. (1943), Individual and mass behavior in extreme conditions. *Amer. J. Abnorm. Soc. Psychol.,* 38:417–453.

Beuchner, H. A. (1986), *Dachau: The Hour of the Avenger; An Eyewitness Account.* Metairie, LA: Thunderbird Press.

Blos, P. (1962), *On Adolescence: A Psychoanalytic Interpretation.* New York: Free Press.

——— (1974), The genealogy of the ego ideal. *The Psychoanalytic Study of the Child,* 29:43–48. New Haven, CT: Yale University Press.

Bremner, J. D., Scott, T. M., Delaney, R. C., Southwick, S. M., Mason, J. W., Johnson, D. R., Innis, S. B., McCarthy, G., & Charney, D. S. (1993), Deficits in short-term memory in posttraumatic stress disorder. *Amer. J. Psychiat.,* 150:1015–1019.

Carmil, D., & Carel, R. S. (1986), Emotional distress and satisfaction in life among Holocaust survivors—A community study of survivors and controls. *Psycholog. Med.,* 16:141–149.

Cohen, E. A. (1953), *Human Behavior in the Concentration Camp.* New York: W. W. Norton.

Danieli, Y. (1982), Families of survivors and the Nazi Holocaust. Some short and long-term effects. *Stress and Anxiety,* 8:405–423. Washington, DC: Hemisphere.

Dasberg, H. (1987), Psychological distress of Holocaust survivors and offspring in Israel forty years later: A review. *Israel J. Psychiat. & Rel. Sci.,* 24:245–256.

Davidson, S. (1979), Massive psychic traumatization and social support. *J. Psychosom. Res.,* 23:395–402.

———— (1980), The clinical effects of massive psychic trauma in families of Holocaust survivors. *J. Marit. & Fam. Therapy,* 6:11–21.

———— (1985), Group formation and its significance in the Nazi concentration camps. *Israel J. Psychiat. & Rel. Sci.,* 22:41–50.

Des Pres, T. (1976), *The Survivor.* New York: Oxford.

Eissler, K. R. (1967), Perverted psychiatry. *Amer. J. Psychiatry,* 123:1352–1358.

Eitinger, L. (1961), Pathology of the concentration camp syndrome. *Arch. Gen. Psychiatry,* 5:371–377.

Engdahl, B. E., Harkness, A. R., Eberly, R. E., Page, N. F., & Brelinski, J. (1993), Structural models of captivity trauma, resilience, and trauma response among former prisoners of war 20 to 40 years after release. *Soc. Psychiatry Psychiatric Epidemiol.,* 28:109–115.

Fleming, J., & Altschul, S. (1963), Activation of mourning and growth by psychoanalysis. *Internat. J. Psycho-Anal.,* 44:419–431.

Frankl, V. E. (1959), *Man's Search for Meaning.* New York: Simon & Schuster.

Friedman, P. (1949), Some aspects of concentration camp psychology. *Amer. J. Psychiatry,* 105:601–605.

Gilbert, M. (1996), *The Boys.* London: Weidenfeld & Nicolson.

Grubrich-Simitis, I. (1981), Extreme traumatization as cumulative trauma. *The Psychoanalytic Study of the Child,* 36:415–450. New Haven, CT: Yale University Press.

———— (1984), From concretism to metaphor. *The Psychoanalytic Study of the Child,* 39:301–319. New Haven, CT: Yale University Press.

Hoppe, K. D. (1967), The emotional reactions of psychiatrists confronting survivors of persecution. *Psychoanal. Forum,* 3:187–196.

Jacobson, E. (1965), The return of the lost parent. In: *Drives, Affects and Behavior,* Vol. 2, ed. M. Schur. New York: International Universities Press, pp. 193–211.

Kahana, B., Harel, Z., & Kahana, E. (1988), Predictors of psychological well-being among survivors of the Holocaust. In: *Human Adaptation to Extreme Stress,* ed. J. P. Wilson, Z. Harel, & B. Kahana. New York: Plenum.

Klein, H. (1973), Children of the Holocaust. Mourning and bereavement. In: *The Child in His Family, The Impact of Disease and Death,* ed. E. J. Anthony & C. Koupernick. New York: Wiley.

———— Zellermayer, J., & Shanan, J. (1963), Former concentration camp inmates on a psychiatric ward. *Arch. Gen. Psychiatry,* 8:334–342.

Koenig, N. (1964), Chronic or persisting identity diffusion. *Amer. J. Psychiatry,* 120:1081–1084.

Krell, R. (1990), Holocaust survivors: A clinical perspective. *Psychiat. J. Univ. Ottawa,* 15:18–21.

Kris, E. (1944), Art and regression. *NY Acad. Sci.,* 6:236–250.

Krystal, H., & Niederland, W. G. (1968), Clinical observations on the survivor syndrome. In: *Massive Psychic Trauma,* ed. H. Krystal. New York: International Universities Press.

Kuch, K., & Cox, B. J. (1992), Symptoms of PTSD in 123 survivors of the Holocaust. *Amer. J. Psychiatry,* 149:337–340.

Leon, G. R., Butcher, J. N., Kleinman, M., Goldberg, A., & Almagor, M. (1981), Survivors of the Holocaust and their children: Current status and adjustment. *J. Personal. Soc. Psychol.,* 41:503–516.

Levi, P. (1969), *Survival in Auschwitz.* New York: Collier.

Lifton, R. J. (1972), Questions of guilt. *Partisan Rev.,* 39:514–530.

Major, E. E. (1996), The impact of the Holocaust on the second generation: Norwegian Jewish Holocaust survivors and their children. *J. Traumat. Stress,* 9:441–444.

Mant, A. K. (1978), Genocide. *J. Foren. Sci. Soc.,* 18:13–17.

Marrus, M. R. (1985), *The Holocaust in History.* London: University Press of New England.

Matussek, P. (1975), *Internment in Concentration Camps and Its Consequences.* New York: Springer-Verlag.

Nadler, A., & Ben-Shushan, D. (1989), Forty years later: Long term consequences of massive traumatization as manifested by Holocaust survivors from the city and the kibbutz. *J. Consult. & Clin. Psychol.,* 57:287–293.

Niederland, W. G. (1968), Clinical observations on the "Survivor Syndrome." *Internat. J. Psycho-Anal.,* 49:313–315.

Pedersen, S. (1948), Psychopathological reactions to extreme social displacements. *Psychoanal. Rev.,* 35:344–354.

Pennebaker, J. W., Barger, J. S. D., & Tiebout, J. (1989), Disclosure of traumas among Holocaust survivors. *Psychosom. Med.,* 51:577–589.

Pollak, R. (1997), *The Creation of Dr. B.* New York: Simon & Schuster.

Prescott, D. T. (1986), Reflections of forty years ago—Belsen 1945. *J. Roy. Army Med. Corps,* 132:48–51.

Rakoff, V., Sigal, J. J., & Epstein, N. B. (1967), Children and families of concentration camp survivors. *Can. Ment. Health,* 14:24–26.

Robins, S., Rapport-Bar-Sever, M., & Rapport, J. (1994), The present state of people who survived the Holocaust as children. *Acta Psychiatr. Scand.,* 89:242–245.

Ryn, Z. (1986), Suicides in the Nazi concentration camps. *Suicide & Life-Threat. Behav.,* 16:419–433.

———— (1990), The evolution of mental disturbances in the concentration camp syndrome (K-Z syndrome). *Genet. Soc. Gen. Psychol. Monog.,* 116:21–36.

Solkoff, N. (1992), Children of survivors of the Nazi Holocaust: A critical review of the literature. *Amer. J. Orthopsychiat.,* 62:342–358.

Southwick, S. M., Yehuda, R., & Giller, E. L. (1993), Personality disorders in treatment-seeking combat veterans with post-traumatic stress disorder. *Amer. J. Psychiatry,* 150:1020–1023.

Speed, N., Engdahl, B. E., Schwartz, J., & Eberly, R. E. (1989), Posttraumatic stress disorder as a consequence of the prisoner of war experience. *J. Posttraum. Ment. Dis.,* 177:147–153.

Stavroulakis, N. P., & DeVinney, T. J. (1992), *Jewish Sites and Synagogues of Greece.* Athens: Talos Press.

Sterba, E. (1968), The effects of persecution on adolescents. In: *Massive Psychic Trauma,* ed. H. Krystal. New York: International Universities Press.

Sugar, M. (1968), Normal adolescent mourning. *Amer. J. Psychother.*, 22:258–269.

——— (1988), A preschooler in a disaster. *Amer. J. Psychother.*, 42:619–629.

——— (1990a), Developmental anxieties in adolescence. *Adol. Psychiatry,* 17:385–403.

——— Ed. (1990b), *Atypical Adolescence and Sexuality.* New York: Norton.

Sutker, P. B., Winstead, D. K., Galina, Z. H., & Allain, A. N. (1991), Cognitive deficits and psychopathology among former prisoners of war and combat veterans of the Korean conflict. *Amer. J. Psychiatry,* 148:67–72.

Thygesen, P. (1980), The concentration camp syndrome. *Dan. Med. Bull.*, 27:224–228.

Times-Picayune (1995), April 12: A1.

Trautman, E. C. (1971), Violence and victims in Nazi concentration camps and the psychopathology of the survivors. *Internat. Psychiat. Clin.*, 87:115–133.

Werner, E. E., & Smith, R. S. (1982), *Vulnerable but Invincible.* New York: McGraw-Hill.

Winnicott, D. W. (1957), The antisocial tendency. In: *Collected Papers, Through Paediatrics to Psychoanalysis.* New York: Basic Books.

Wolfenstein, M. (1966), How is mourning possible? *The Psychoanalytic Study of the Child,* 21:93–123. New York: International Universities Press.

Yehuda, R., Kahana, B., Southwick, S. M., & Giller, E. L. (1994), Depressive features in Holocaust survivors with post-traumatic stress disorder. *J. Traum. Stress,* 7:699–704.

Author Index

Subject Index